The Ultimate Self-Help Guide for MEN

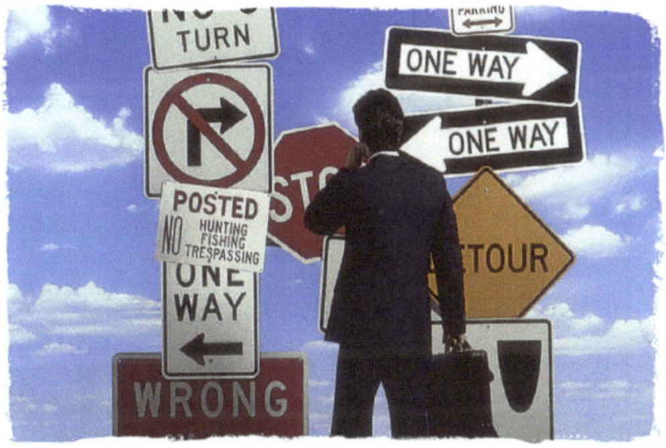

Joe Novella

Produced by Words and Webs 2012 edition
www.wordsandwebs.com.au
info@wordsandwebs.com.au

Originally published 2006

All of the characters in this book are fictitious and any resemblance to actual people, living or dead, is purely coincidental.

Novella, Joe

The Ultimate Self-Help Guide for Men
ISBN: 978-0-9871844-3-6
pp288

About the Author

Joe was born and raised in Melbourne, Australia. After graduating from high school he began studying for a Computer Science degree, and looked set for a lucrative career in the IT industry and a comfortable middle-class life in the 'burbs'. But IT was not for him, so he dropped out of university and took off overseas. His plan was to use his part-time bar work experience as a passport to working his way around the world, broadening his horizons, sowing his wild oats, and hopefully gaining some insight as to what he should do with his life along the way.

Ten years later, after working in one pub after another, in one country after another, Joe arrived back in Australia. Though he was still no wiser as to his life's purpose, he was much wiser in life—on account of his many and varied cultural travel experiences, of which he lists Oktoberfest in Germany, a visit to the Guinness factory in Ireland, and some church with a painted ceiling in Italy as the highlights.

Joe now works as a barman at an inner-city pub, a job he has held for the past two years. According to him, he spends as much time drawing on his wisdom to counsel unhappy men as he does pulling beers. And in so doing, it suddenly dawned on him that his purpose in life is to help his fellow man—not just those who visit the pub, but all men. And so he decided to write a self-help book—not just any self-help book, but the *ultimate* self-help book.

What qualifies Joe to write such a book? The answer—life experience. Joe may not have any formal qualifications, or fancy letters after his name, but what he does have is an Honours Degree from the University of Life.

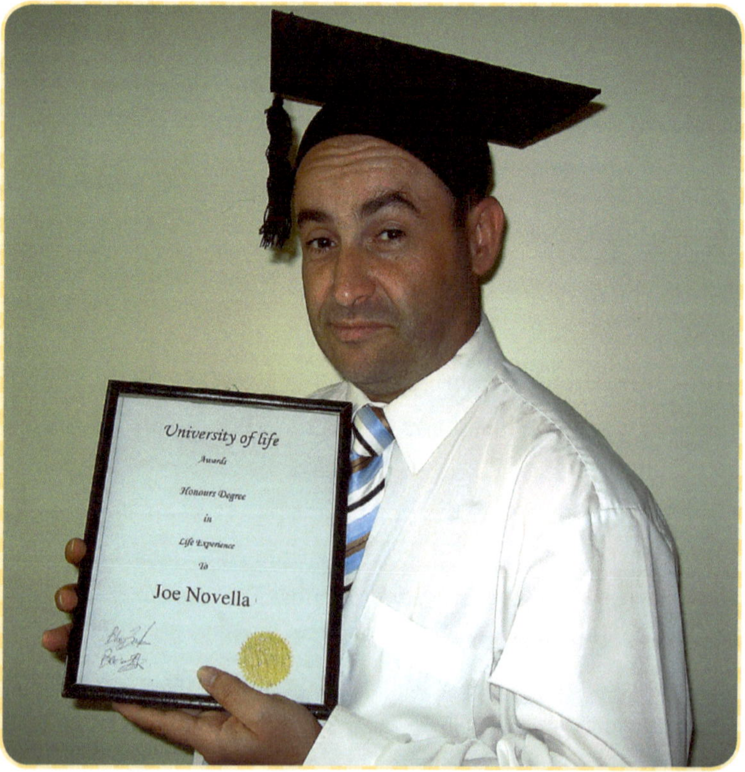

Acknowledgements

To the many friends who volunteered their minds and bodies for this project, I thank you and hope you enjoyed making the book happen as much as I did.

Contents

Introduction 1

Part I — Understanding ourselves 5

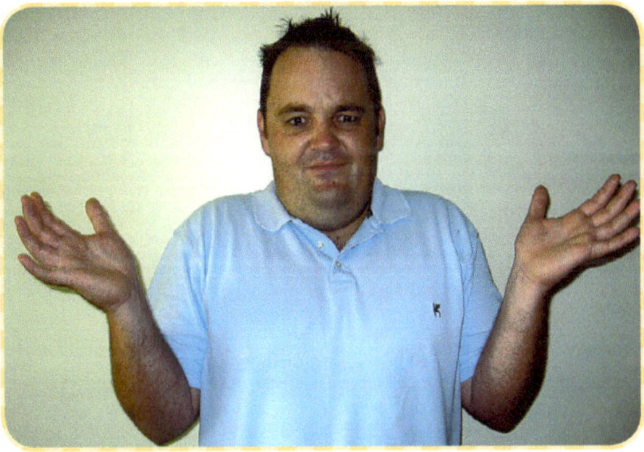

Chapter 1 Men in the modern world 7

Chapter 2 Rediscovering what makes us men 9

Chapter 3 Learn to love your penis 11

Chapter 4 Rediscovering the inner child 17

Chapter 5 Every man needs a shed 21

Chapter 6 Redefining what it means to be a successful man 25

Part II — The wonderful mystery that is Woman 33

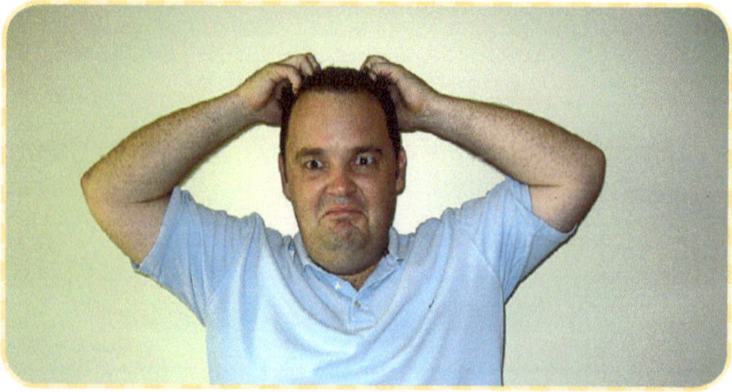

Chapter 7 Understanding women 35
Chapter 8 She is not your mum 41
Chapter 9 What women really want from their men 43

Part III — Successfully single 51

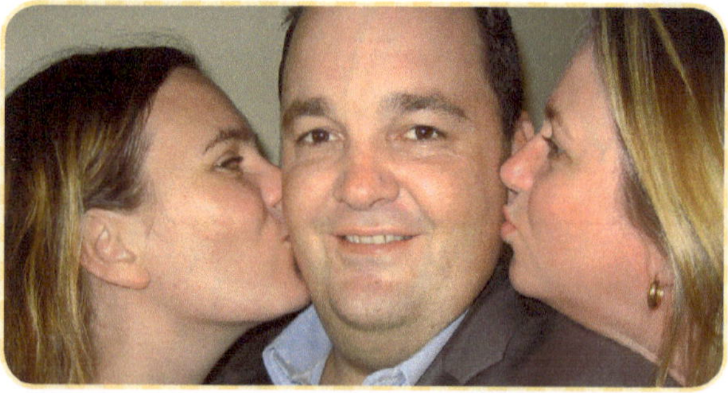

Chapter 10 Why are there so many unhappy singles out there? 53
Chapter 11 Sowing our wild oats successfully 57
Chapter 12 How to get lucky, even if you're ugly 63
Chapter 13 Understanding our competition 65
Chapter 14 Location, location, location 69
Chapter 15 It's all about advertising 73
Chapter 16 Reeling them in 77
Chapter 17 Internet dating success 87
Chapter 18 A single man's guide to sex 93

Part IV — Starting a relationship 103

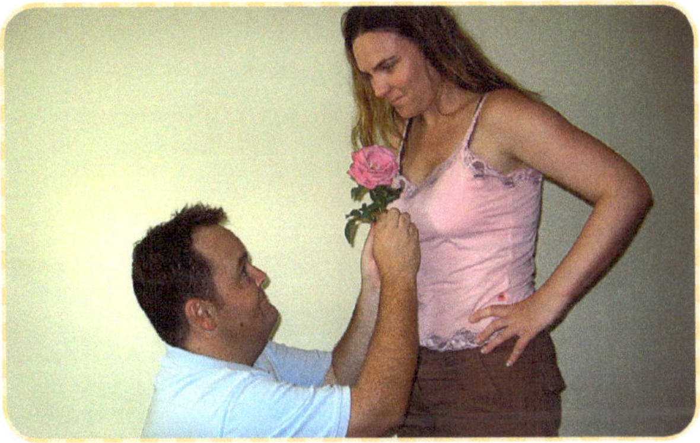

Chapter 19 Am I ready for a steady girlfriend? 105
Chapter 20 Winning her over 109

Part V — Fat and happy: The science of successful long-term relationships 119

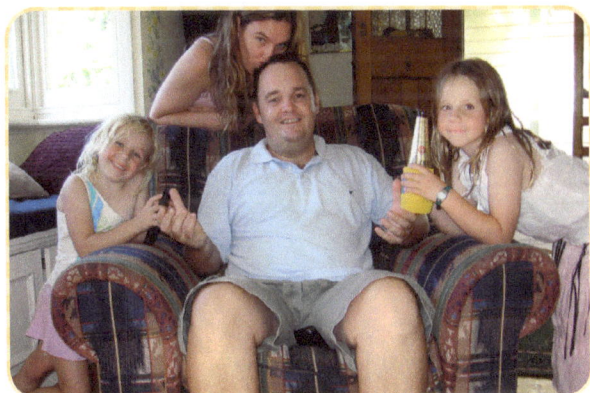

Chapter 21 Warning: There's a huge difference between a girlfriend and a wife 121
Chapter 22 Why do so many long-term relationships fail? 127
Chapter 23 Why do relationships succeed? 133
Chapter 24 Wearing the pants 137

Chapter 25	Learning to avoid conflict	141
Chapter 26	The magical 'leave pass'	145
Chapter 27	Getting out of the dog house	155
Chapter 28	Making sure she only has eyes for you	159
Chapter 29	Sex for men in long-term relationships	165

Part VI — Looking good, feeling great, living well 177

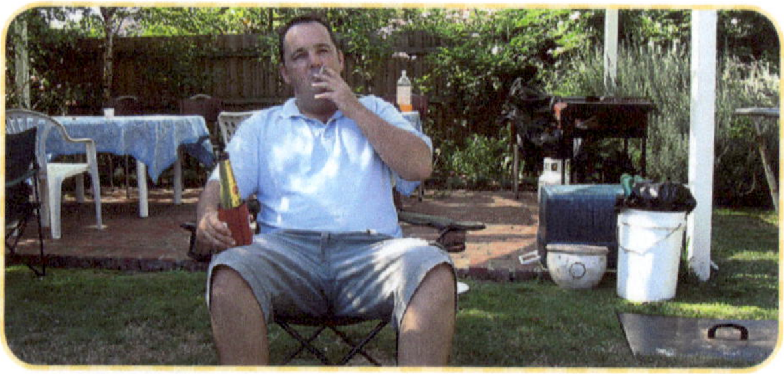

Introduction		179
Chapter 30	Grooming	181
Chapter 31	Diet and exercise	189
Chapter 32	A healthy mind	195
Chapter 33	First aid for common male ailments	199

Part VII — A user's guide to alcohol 205

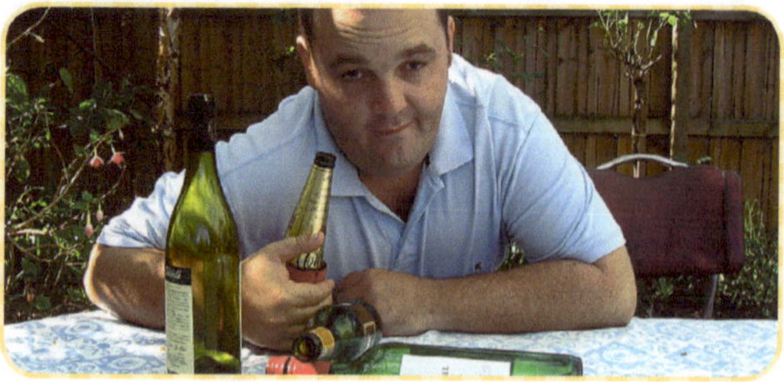

Chapter 34	Know your poison	207
Chapter 35	Alcohol and status	211
Chapter 36	Traps for young players	215

Chapter 37 Hangovers 223
Chapter 38 Other unwanted by-products of a night out on the turps 227
Chapter 39 The step-by-step guide to handling your drink 233

Great drinks for a top night out 237

Part VIII — Everyday hints and tips 241

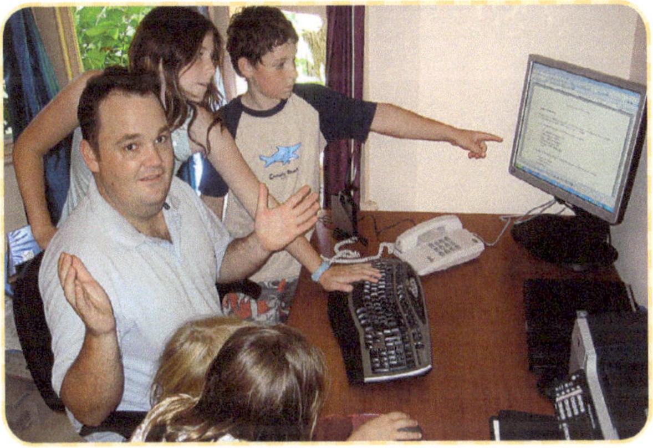

Chapter 40 A man's guide to using a PC 243
Chapter 41 How to handle yourself in a punch-on 251
Chapter 42 The lost art of the fart 261
Chapter 43 Social etiquette for the average Joe 267

The final word 273

Introduction

Why do we need another self-help book when the world is full of them?

The answer—because the other self-help books out there don't understand what is really important to us men; they don't understand what makes us happy. They are full of psychological mumbo-jumbo, full of unreal people with unreal stories, and recommendations that are way too hard to put into action.

What's so different about this self-help book?

The answer—it offers real-life solutions to real-life problems. Us men don't want to sit on our bums discovering our inner selves. We don't want to spend time learning to deal with our emotions, or listening to our partners while they deal with theirs. We want shortcuts and ready-made answers to everyday challenges; answers that require bugger-all effort and little or no time. We want to know practical stuff, like how we can get a weekend away with our mates and not feel guilty; how we can fart in bed without pissing off the missus; how to avoid giving cuddles and foot massages, or at least how to use them to our advantage; and how to make women think we're sex gods even if we're not.

What makes me such an expert?

I'm not. In order to produce a well-rounded, knowledge-packed text, I have complemented my own expertise with input from the hundreds of men I have met whilst attending family or social functions, travelling overseas and working in my current job at the pub. The men I have consulted are from many different walks of life, and include doctors, lawyers, scientists, plumbers, as well as poets and pissed idiots. They are fathers, sons, brothers and lovers. Together they have taught me what works and what doesn't work when it comes to the pursuit of happiness—and you, the reader, will be the beneficiary of their experience.

Where is the professionalism, the science?

Though I work at the pub of a night, during the day I attend courses at the local college, in subjects such as *DP101 — Digital Photography: From NO to PRO in one week*, and *PW201 — Power Writing: Wow them with quotes and jargon*—all to give the book the high level of professionalism and polish the modern-day reader demands. I have also enlisted the help of some of the academics who visit the pub on a regular basis (before they get too drunk) to help verify the formulae, graphs, tables and diagrams that I use to explain some of the more complex ideas. I'm sure you'll be impressed.

So, without further ado, get ready to become happier, healthier, more worldly, and irresistible to women.

Please enjoy,
Joe, the author
PHD, MVP, LMFAO, ROFL — Life Studies

PART I

Understanding ourselves

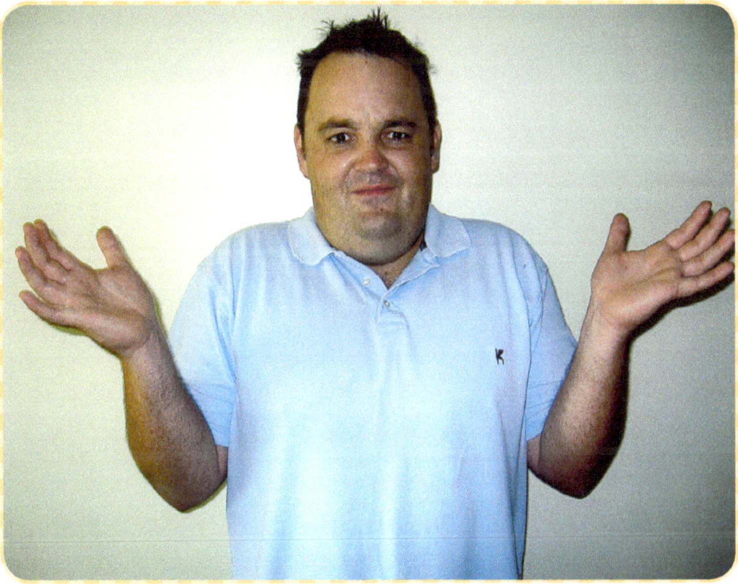

Chapter 1
Men in the modern world

Let's face it, most blokes these days don't know if they're from Venus, Mars or hitching a ride on some out of control comet heading straight for a black hole. Life for us men was much more straightforward a few decades ago, when we knew who we were and what was expected of us. We brought home the bacon, mowed the lawn, washed the dog, changed flat tyres and made decisions. We were protectors, providers, fathers, lovers and brothers. We were men.

But times have changed, and the concept of 'manhood' is no longer clear. Defining the 'modern man' has become a stoush involving many combatants. In one corner we have the old-timers telling us how "men were men" in the old days, and how we should follow their lead; in the other corner we have the mass media—films, magazines, radio and advertisers—telling us what it means to be a successful modern man. In yet another corner we have our partners and girlfriends, who are no longer afraid to demand more of us as men, and who will no longer settle for a P&P (Penis and Pay check) type of guy.

In short, everyone is telling us how to be men. There are so many mixed messages on manhood, so many different points of view, that we are no longer sure what is right and what is wrong. Is a man who stays at home to look after the kids while the wife earns a crust less of a man than a captain of industry on a huge wage and his 3rd wife? Should we spend as much time on our grooming and on learning how to express our emotions as we do in the garage, garden or shed? We have lost the knowledge of what truly makes us men. We are confused. We have become insecure in our manhood and, ultimately, many of us are unhappy.

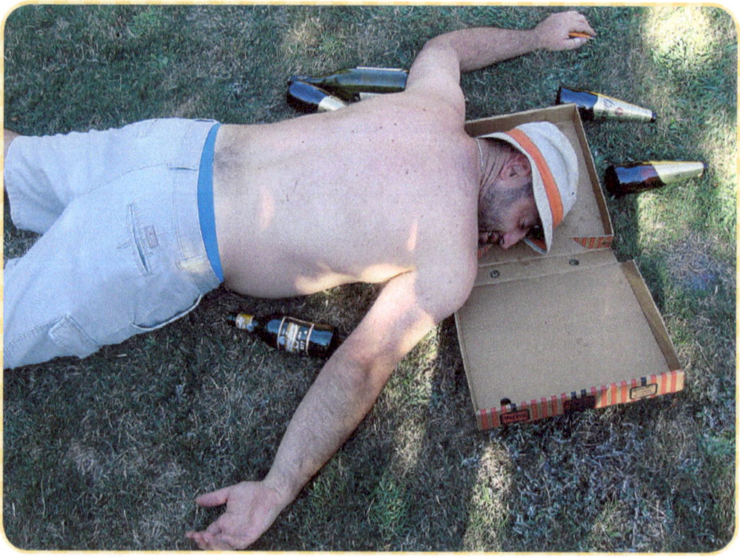

The modern man — unhappy, confused and insecure.

How do we reverse this trend towards confusion and unhappiness? We start by rediscovering the true meaning of what it means to be a man. How do we do that? Read on.

Chapter 2
Rediscovering what makes us men

A billion-dollar industry has been created to service the insecure and confused man. There are bucket-loads of books, workshops and courses available, all aimed at helping us men rediscover our manhood. GUYS, DON'T WASTE YOUR MONEY! No amount of expensive clothes, hair products, 'back-sack-and-crack waxes' or weekends away beating drums to rediscover the warrior within will ever make us happy in the long term. Don't get me wrong, all the above products and activities are important for our self-esteem, but until we become comfortable with the very essence of our manhood they will only provide short-term gain.

What is the very essence of manhood? To answer this question we must strip away everything that we have heard, read or been told about what it is to be a man, and go back to the core. Let us think of ourselves as onions. The outer layers are how we identify ourselves to society: our jobs, houses, wives, girlfriends, cars, clothes and so on. The outer layers consist of the material symbols of manhood. Strip these away and we begin to see ourselves in less material terms, as providers, nurturers, defenders and protectors. Continue to strip away the layers until we get to the core, and what are we left with? A PENIS!

That's right. Forget all the airy-fairy stuff about being a man, the indisputable characteristic that makes us men is our penis, and the sooner we get a grip on this the quicker we'll learn to become secure in our manhood.

Chapter 3
Learn to love your penis

What man needs fame or fortune
if he is hung like a donkey?
(Source — An old West Indian proverb)

Now that we have stripped ourselves back to our core and have rediscovered what it truly means to be a man, we can start rebuilding the layers that will redefine our sense of manhood; layers that will lead to security in our identity and result in sustainable happiness. Learning to love your penis is the first and most fundamental layer we need to add. I like to call this step the 'quest for PPI' (Positive Penis Image). PPI simply means reconnecting with the essence of our manhood, becoming friends with it, and loving it unconditionally no matter what shape or size it is.

What if we don't like our penis?

Recently I surveyed the patrons at the pub with the simple question: Are you happy with your penis? The response was a resounding "yes". I then asked another question: If a magical genie popped out of your beer can and said that he could give you a bigger penis, without the pain of surgery and without anybody else knowing, would you accept it? Once again the answer was a resounding "yes". This simple survey demonstrates that 99.9% of men do not have a PPI. In fact, this is the root cause of all our self-esteem problems.

Us men, quite incorrectly, equate penis size with power and potency. When we're not happy with the size of our penis, our PPI suffers and we spend our whole lives trying to compensate. I call this phenomenon 'Napoleon's conundrum'. In other words: the smaller the penis, the greater the need to overcompensate. The conundrum lies in the fact that no matter how much we overcompensate, we will never truly be happy. Napoleon is a good example because he demonstrates that it's no good ruling the world if you're not happy with your member and your lady bursts out laughing every time you drop your strides.

Napoleon's conundrum

$$E = 1/S$$

Where E (Overcompensation Energy Expenditure) is inversely proportional to S (Size of Penis).

The formula was hit upon after a particularly long afternoon session with neighbour Dave. Turns out Dave was a bit of a maths wiz in his younger days, and the photo below is of him demonstrating the finer points of the formula using an estimation of his own penis size to explain why he's such a laid-back character with no need to overcompensate.

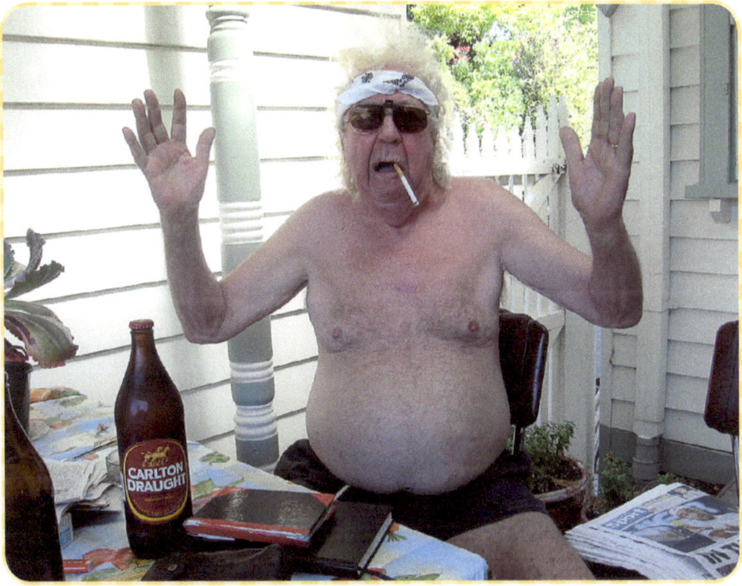

How do we achieve PPI?

Let's face it, if all us men were hung like John Holmes then it wouldn't matter if we were balding, lard-arsed couch potatoes—we'd all be bullet-proof. But we're not all hung like JH, so how do we achieve PPI even if we're a little short-changed in the size department? We could go out and get surgically enhanced, or buy a mail-order product from a Scandinavian country; but that costs money, and the results aren't always desirable. I mean, who wants to risk their penis looking like an inflated porcupine fish as a result of botched surgery or a faulty pump device? No, there is a much easier way to achieve PPI, and here's how:

1. Extension by distention

(distention: the act of being stretched, inflated)

If we're on the small side of average south of the belt buckle, and we're sick of the lads down at the footy club having a laugh at our expense every time we hit the showers, or our girlfriend saying stuff like, "Don't worry, honey, it's not big but it's cute", then why not try the following simple but effective technique:

> ***A simple technique:*** The next time you're down at the footy club preparing to hit the showers, or at home preparing for a romantic night in with the missus, drink a litre of water 15 minutes before undressing. You'll be pleasantly surprised to find your penis looking like an engorged cucumber. Swagger into those showers, or into the bedroom, like an outlawed gun-slinger, with your cucumber proudly swinging in the breeze. And nobody, but nobody, will ever laugh at you again.

2. Personify your penis — give it a name

Giving our penis a name establishes a relationship between it and us. As a result, it ceases to be simply an appendage and takes on a personality all of its own. Imagine a flea-infested, three-legged dog limping past us in the street. We feel sorry for it, but we move on. Now imagine if that same three-legged dog had a name. All of a sudden the dog has a personality we can empathise with, and we're likely to bend down and pat it. Imagine if our partner is with us: she is likely to bend down and pat it as well. If little Johnny from across the road starts laughing at the dog, then our partner is likely to say, "Hey, little Johnny, you leave Fido alone—he may have fleas and three legs but he's beautiful all the same." The same applies to our penis.

An advanced technique: Rather than give your penis an ordinary name—like Joe, Ted or Bill—give it an exotic name. I like to use Spanish or Italian names, like Federico or Fernando, Rosario or Don Juan. The Spanish and Italians are renowned for their passion, and the womenfolk go weak at the knees at the thought of shagging some handsome, hot-blooded Valentino. Plus, using a Spanish or Italian name for your penis will make you feel as though you're packing a Latino-love-god between your legs, and, consequently, your self-esteem will skyrocket.

Chapter 4
Rediscovering the inner child

Man-child, Man-child, Man-child,
Where have you gone?
Why have you forsaken me like a tennis ball hit over the fence?
Or a prized sausage that's rolled off the BBQ?
Lost like the pets of my youth that grew old and were sent by my parents to that mysterious farm from which they never returned.
(Source: Amateur poets' corner —
Thursday nights at the Pier Hotel)

Meet little Jono

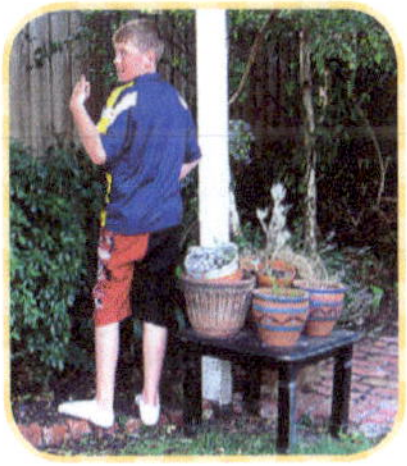

Why is little Jono peeing on his mother's newly-planted garden bed? He has no idea. Being a kid means he doesn't need a reason for his actions.

It also means he is unable to explain his actions when his mum asks, "What's wrong with using the toilet, Jono?" The best he can offer is a shrug of his shoulders and the observation, "I don't know, Mum, I just felt like it." Is Jono happy, despite having no good reason to pee on the snapdragons? Of course he is.

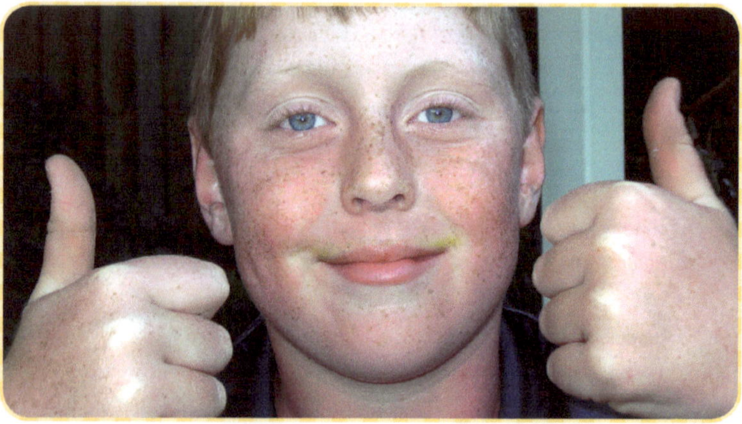

There is a little Jono living inside every one of us. Unfortunately, as we grow older the little Jono is either lost, as we try to conform to society's expectations regarding what it means to be a man, or beaten out of us in an attempt to ensure that we grow up to be mature, responsible men.

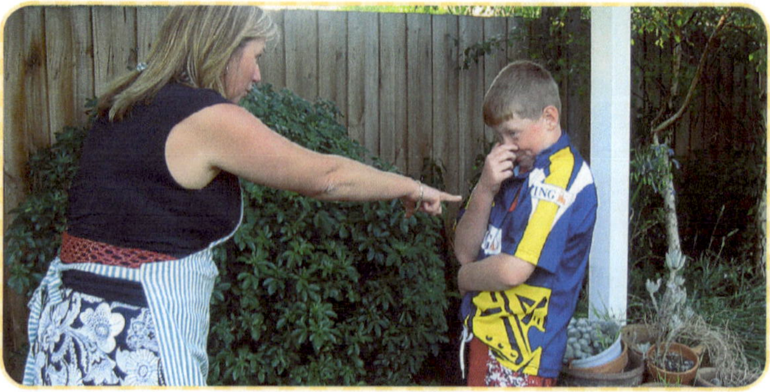

At some point in our lives, we men need to rediscover our inner little Jono. This process of rediscovery is the next layer we need to add on our journey to becoming happier men. And it's not that hard to do. It's all about remembering the joy of doing something for no reason at all—something a little crazy, something that's just for fun—and then going off and doing it.

How do we rediscover our little Jono? We perform what I like to term 'acts of liberation'. Whether it be running around the village of a ski resort naked (a personal favourite of mine) or going to a meeting at work dressed as one of the Village People (only advisable if you are the boss), us men will be genuinely surprised at how good acts of liberation can make us feel.

Takeaway learning: Men are happiest when they are able to do things for no good reason except for a laugh. It reminds them that life is an adventure, that they are king of the world and master of their domain.

Suggested acts of liberation

- Collect the mail wearing nothing but a pair of gumboots.
- Buy yourself a crazy pet, like an eel or a donkey.
- Go for a skinny-dip in your neighbour's pool.

Remember—the older us men get, the more society places restraints on our behaviour, and we can end up feeling trapped and restricted as a result. It's up to us to break the bonds.

Chapter 5
Every man needs a shed

In man-talk, 'shed' is another way of saying personal space. A place where we can go and shut out the world for a little while and be at one with ourselves. The need for our own personal space is part of our makeup, and it starts from a very early age. Take little Timmy, for example.

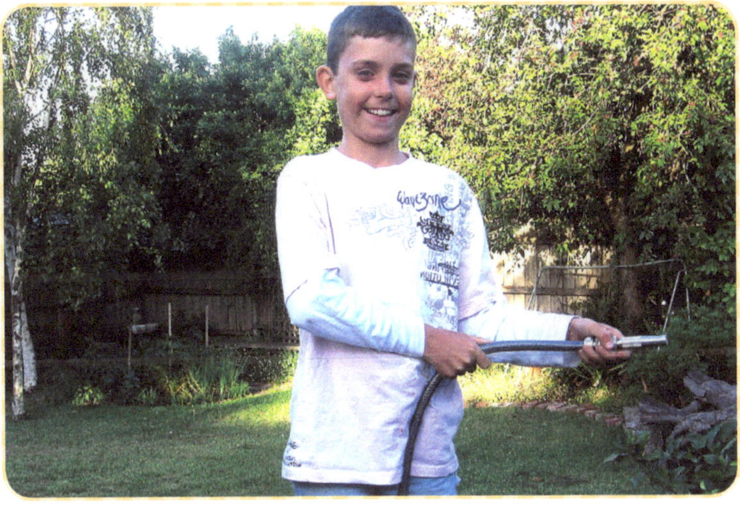

On first inspection of the photo below, we're likely to think of Timmy as a renegade kid who needs a good swift kick up the backside. But when we investigate his motives a little deeper, we understand that all Timmy is trying to do is establish and protect his own personal space (in this instance, the trampoline).

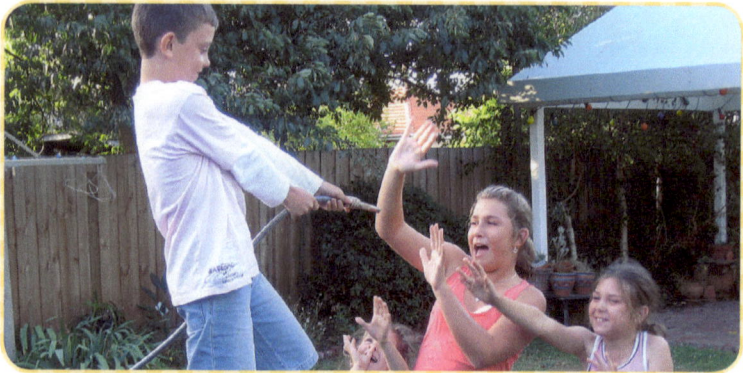

How does Timmy feel after winning his battle? The answer — like a champion.

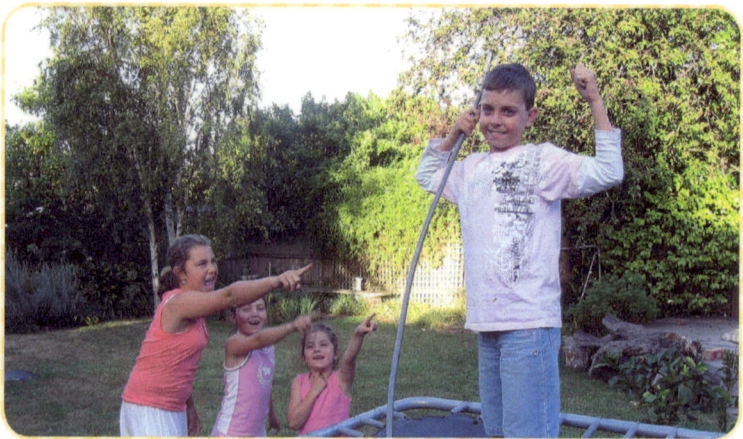

As adults, the need for our own personal and private space increases. We need a place where we can read the paper or have a little nap. But establishing our own personal space can be difficult, and there are often repercussions.

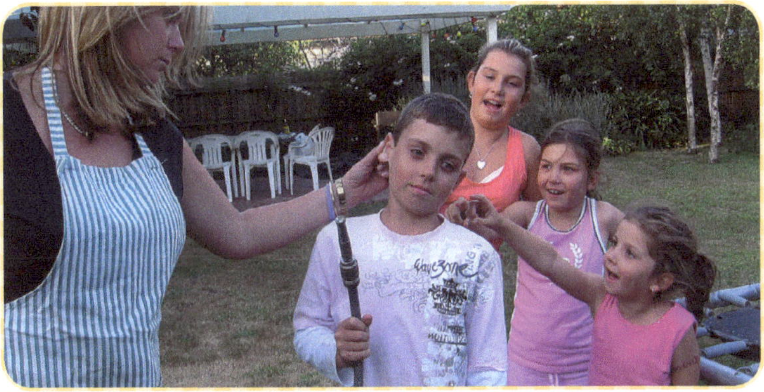

Women are mystified as to why us men spend so long in the toilet. We do this because, for most of us, there's probably no other place in the house where we can get some peace and quiet. It's probably the only place where we can truly be alone, and it's also where most of us do our best thinking.

However, us men need more than just the toilet as our personal space haven, because sure enough, just like clockwork, every time we get in there everyone else in the household will suddenly feel the urge for a visit. And even if we don't get disturbed, we'll probably end up with a verbal cuff across the head from our partners, when we exit, for stinking the place up and spending so long in there.

So, it is vitally important for our well-being as men to establish a 'me only' zone (unless we want to spend the rest of our lives snatching moments of peace and quiet on the bog). The 'me only' zone may be a shed, a garage, or a room in the house—wherever or whatever it is, we must make it our castle.

Takeaway learning: A man's home may not necessarily be his castle, but a wise man has a castle in his own home.

Chapter 6
Redefining what it means to be a successful man

The most successful man in the world is not necessarily the richest, the most powerful, nor even the most famous. The most successful man in the world is the man who can afford to take an afternoon nap without feeling guilty about it.

(Source: Words of wisdom, printed in English for the benefit of frustrated tourists, underneath the 'CLOSED' sign on the door of a Spanish bank during siesta time)

I wish I had a dollar for every time a bloke has come into the pub feeling more miserable than the miserablest misery guts because he thinks he's a failure. Some of these blokes are truly down and out, without a cent to their name, but most of them are healthy, have a job and a roof over their head. When I remind them of these facts, they respond with, "It's not enough; I want more; I could do better." Why do us men think like this?

The mass media message

Everywhere we look these days—the Internet, movies, billboards, TV and magazines—us blokes are bombarded with images of what it means to be a successful male. Even if we choose to ignore these images, we can bet our bottom dollar that our significant other won't. Believe me, sooner or later we all find ourselves in the situation where we're driving past a billboard showing some well-muscled hunk in Dolce and Gabbana jeans, when our missus leans forward to turn down the volume on the car radio and hits us with, "You know, sweetie, you could do with upgrading your wardrobe."

It's a material world

Madonna was spot-on—we are living in a material world. Factors such as the suburb we live in, how we dress, where we eat, what car we drive and what we do for a living are far more important to those around us than our personality, our character, our values and our dreams. Men these days are trying desperately to keep up with an image, rather than being themselves. It's no wonder most of us are unhappy.

The 'be your best' mentality

Once upon a time it was okay to be average. Not anymore. The evolution of the genus *Beyourbestus Ripeverybodyoffus*—which includes species such as the life coach, the self-improvement guru and the personal trainer—has made it unfashionable to be a Mr Max Mediocre. Throw in the multitude of television shows that teach us men how to dress, cook and furnish our apartments, add a pinch of extreme makeover, and what we have is a pot of 'improve-yourself-or-else' stew.

The net result of all these inputs us men receive from the outside world is an overwhelming pressure to lift our game, or risk being left behind on the scrap heap. And that cannot be healthy.

Laying the foundations for happiness in the modern world

Look, I'm not going to sit here and pretend that being rich, famous, powerful or good-looking won't make us happy, because that's a load of crap. How many ugly poor people do you know who are happy? We'd all like to be rich, famous and so on, but not everyone has what it takes. What us blokes fail to realise is that there are other characteristics of a happy man that are not material in nature and are well within the grasp of all of us.

Experiences count as much as expenses

We don't need to be filthy rich to go camping with our kids. We don't need to be fat-cat company owners to get some real estate for our towels down at the local beach. We'd have more fun touring Europe with 10 mates in an old VW combi than we would in our own private chopper. Experiences are the true currency of happiness. Us men need to treat racking up experiences in the same way we would increasing the bank balance. Experiences create memories, and memories will help cheer us up when we're unwell or down on our luck a lot more than a sackful of cash. Remember, you can't take the Mercedes with you when God comes knocking.

Friendship beats fame and fortune

In the same way that experiences will sustain us through our lives in the good times and the bad, so too will our mates. Having a few good friends is worth much more than a great house in an exclusive neighbourhood.

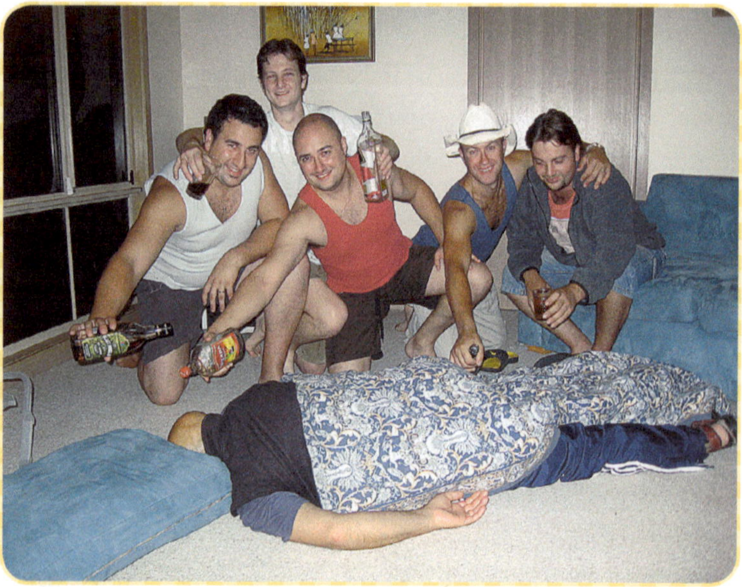

We should never lose sight of the fact that a man with a large circle of friends is wealthy beyond reckoning.

Perspective is power

There are people in this world who are in a bad way and are genuinely in need of help and support; but for the majority of us, things are nearly never as bad as they seem. The ability to have a 'big picture' view of the world gives us the power of perspective, the power to cope with pretty much anything that life throws our way. We may be uglier than a baboon's butt, live in a dog-box flat with 10 other stinky blokes and have a crappy dead-end job; BUT, on the other hand, we *do* have a roof over our head and we definitely won't starve.

Avoid going through life just ticking the boxes

A lot of us blokes feel we have to go through life ticking the boxes: get fit, get better clothes, get wife, get house, get car, get kids, get better job, get makeover, get better house, better car, blah, blah, blah ... By the time we've ticked all the boxes we'll begin to wonder where our lives have gone.

My advice is to slow down and enjoy the moment. We need to take the time to appreciate what's around us, instead of rushing from one milestone to the next. When something special—like falling in love—does happen to us, then we take some time to appreciate the event rather than think, *Okay, what's next?*

> ***Something to ponder:*** Most men only really understand what's important in life when they're facing death, and by then it's too late.

The happiest men are the ones with nothing to prove

Some blokes live their life as if it were one giant competition. They regularly feel the need prove to everyone around them that they're made of the right stuff. They are always competing, and they feel they have to defend their honour every time someone takes even the slightest dig at the way they look or behave.

These kind of blokes may have accumulated substantial assets due to their competitiveness, but they can hardly ever relax. On the other hand, there are blokes out there who couldn't give a hoot about what others think. They don't need the high-powered job or the flashy car, because they don't feel the need to prove anything to anyone. These blokes are usually easygoing, happy, have lots of friends and are unlikely to suffer from stress. Which one would we rather be?

In summary

Fame, fortune and the material trappings that come with them are not the only measure of a successful man. In fact, if I were to create a billboard to epitomise the successful man, one that all us average blokes on the street can aspire to become, the billboard would look something like this:

Be yourself

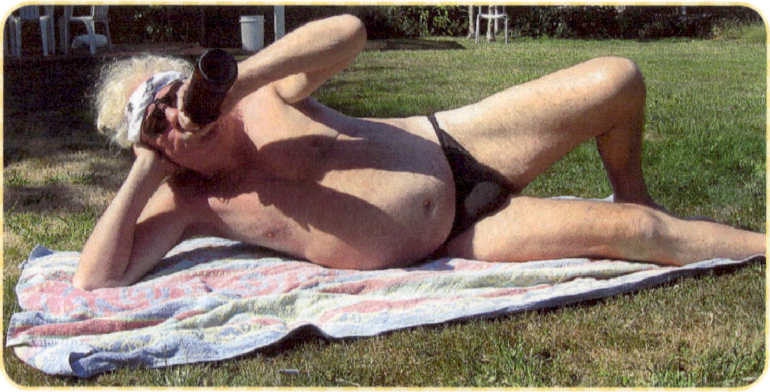

Be happy

Part 1 — Summary and conclusions

Let us think of ourselves as that onion again. The outer layers have been stripped bare, leaving a core of Positive Penis Energy and a fun-loving inner child with nothing to prove—essentially, a man who is well-adjusted and secure in his manhood. The foundation has been set and the basic layers are now in place. It is now time to reconstruct the rest of the layers, in order to rebuild the onion and make it the happiest onion on earth.

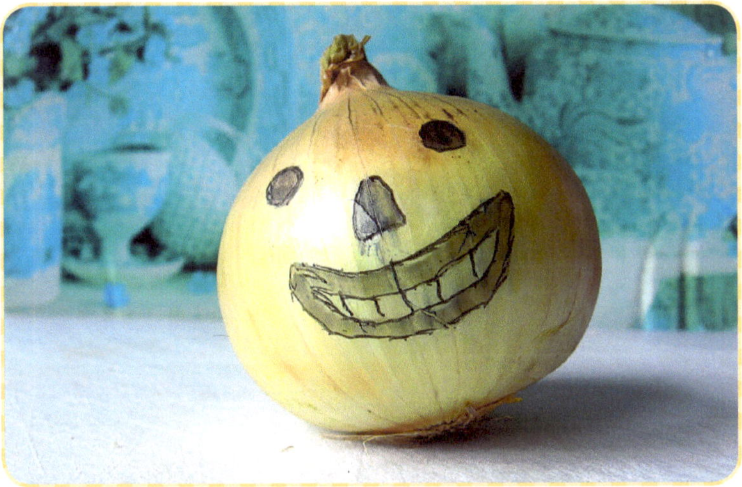

PART II

The wonderful mystery that is Woman

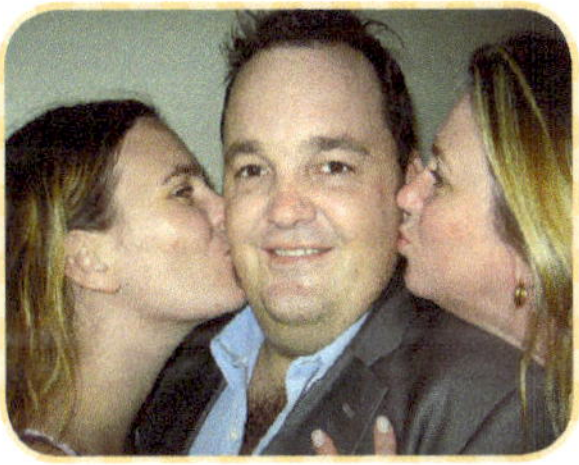

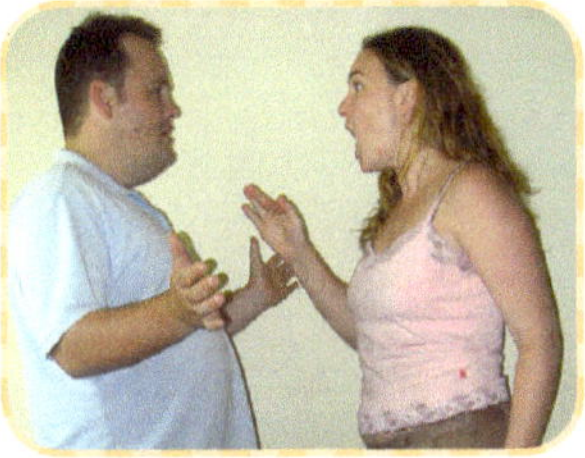

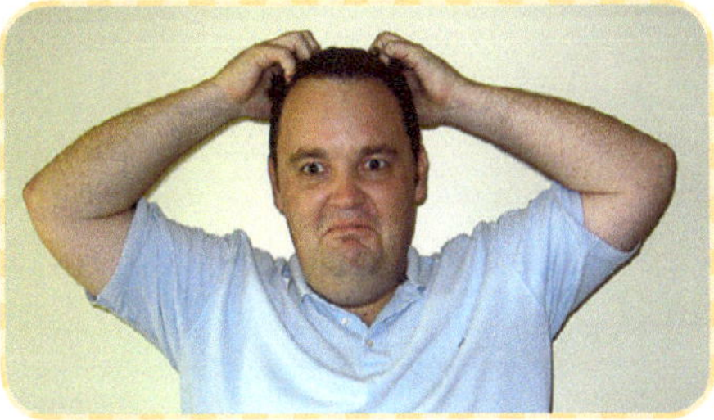

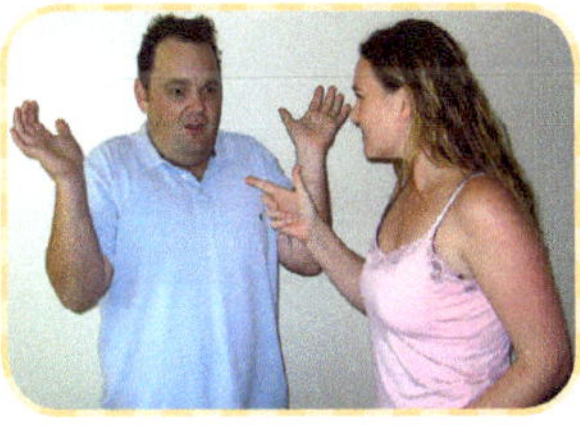

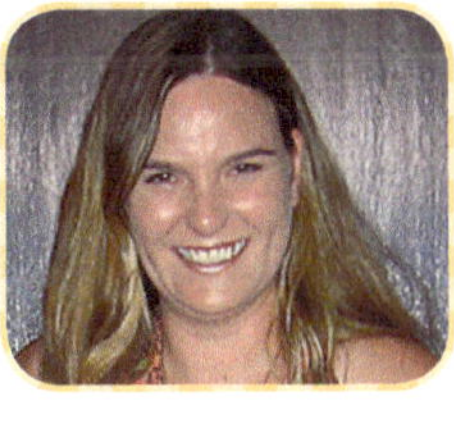

Chapter 7
Understanding women

Adam was sitting around in the Garden of Eden feeling lonely and bored, so he called up to God.

"God, I need someone who will keep me company, understand me, nurture me, excite me and provide me with offspring."

"That will cost you an arm and a leg," God called back.

Adam thought for a moment before replying, "What do I get for a rib?"

Most of us men need women in our lives. They are beautiful, intoxicating, alluring and infuriating—sometimes all at the same time—but our world would be a sad place without them. In fact, our ability to have successful relationships with the opposite sex—whether they be the one-night stand variety or the longer-term commitment type—is one of the most important layers of our identity as men.

One of the steps we must take to ensure our success with women is to try and understand how they work. After all, us men are logical creatures—we like to know how things work before we try to fix them. For example, we can't fix a car if we don't know how the engine works. The problem is, women are not cars, and trying to understand them requires a lot more than just logic.

Top 5 things we know about women but don't understand

(Source: Random survey of drinkers at the pub)

1. They don't always say what they mean or think.
2. They change their minds often.
3. They don't tell us exactly what they want, and get mad when we can't figure it out for ourselves.
4. They sense and feel things about the way we are thinking that are not always correct.
5. They like to get involved in the personal lives of their friends.

Let's face it, ever since the female of the species followed us out of the trees and onto the plains of Africa, us men have been wondering what the hell is going on inside their heads, and we still haven't got a clue. At times they want us to be soft and gentle, to listen and empathise; at others they want us to be strong and direct. They don't want us to give them solutions, yet they get angry when we can't work out how to fix the plumbing. They complain that we can't multi-task, and then get mad when we try doing more than one project at a time (so what if we don't finish any of them?). It's no wonder most of us men don't know if we're Arthur or Martha.

So, how are we meant to have successful relationships with women if we can't work out what's going on inside their heads? Well, one approach is to simply forget about trying to understand them and adopt my mate Louie's philosophy:

Women are like The Matrix *films—don't try and understand them, just enjoy the special effects.*

Using Louie's strategy will avoid a lot of stress but probably won't get us very far in our relationships with women (unless you're rich or famous). In fact, the only women we're likely to form relationships with are the money-exchange variety—table-top dancers, escorts and those whose bedrooms are equipped with webcams.

The truth is, us men will never fully understand the mystery that is woman. But the beauty is, we don't need to. Their mystery is part of their charm. All the female behavioural patterns mentioned above—mind changing, not saying what they think, etc.—are all just symptoms of a far deeper fundamental difference between men and women, and that is, women's sense of reality is different to ours.

***Key point:* Women see the world differently to men**
Us men make the mistake of thinking that women see the world the same way we do—WRONG! We are visual creatures—our reality is what we see. Women's reality is far more complex; it is made up of a mixture of what they see and feel.

A man's reality vs. a woman's reality case study

The following is your typical backyard football finals party. Picture yourself arriving at this party with your partner.

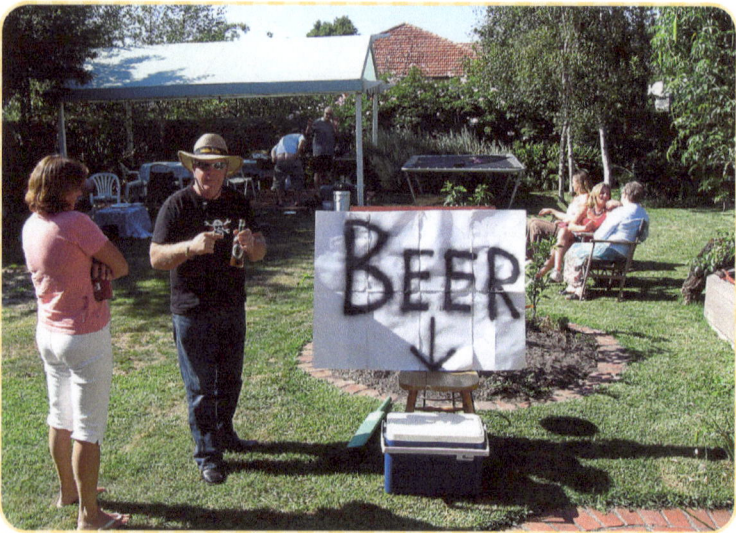

What catches your attention?

You probably notice the BEER sign.

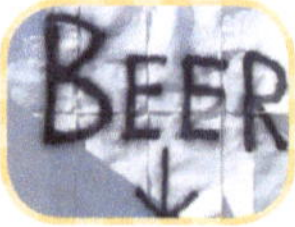

You notice Mick welcoming you with a coldie.

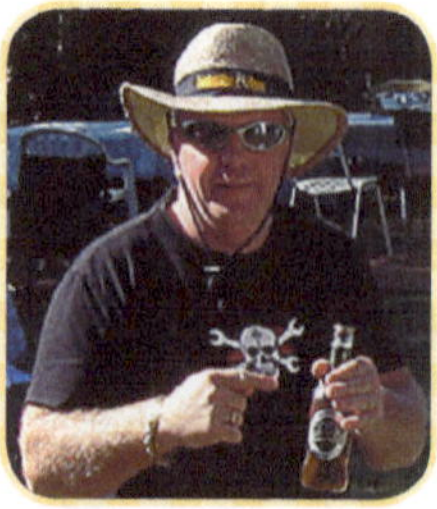

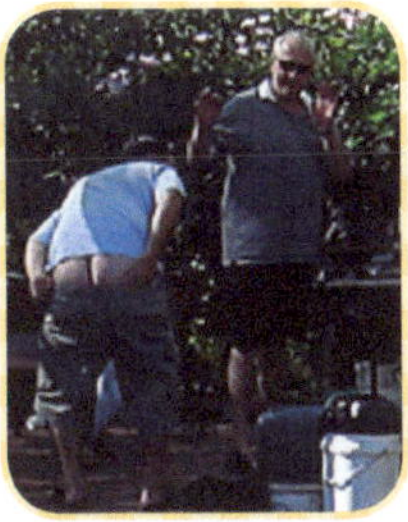

And you have a bit of a laugh when you spot Wayne and Nugget by the BBQ.

What do you think your partner notices?

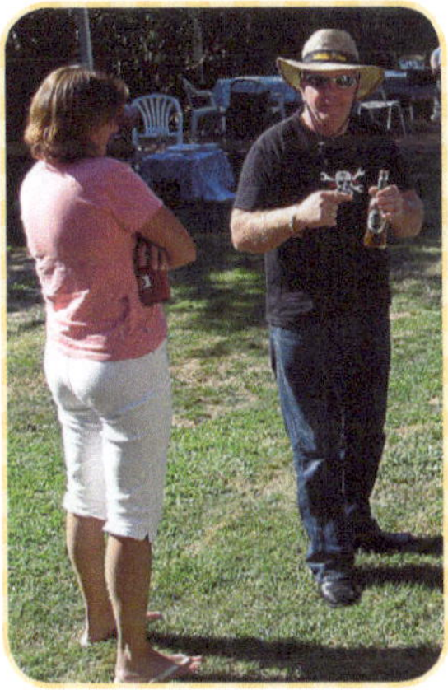

Your partner notices Kerrie looking angry at her husband, Mick. She wonders why Kerry is so angry, and thinks maybe they are having relationship issues.

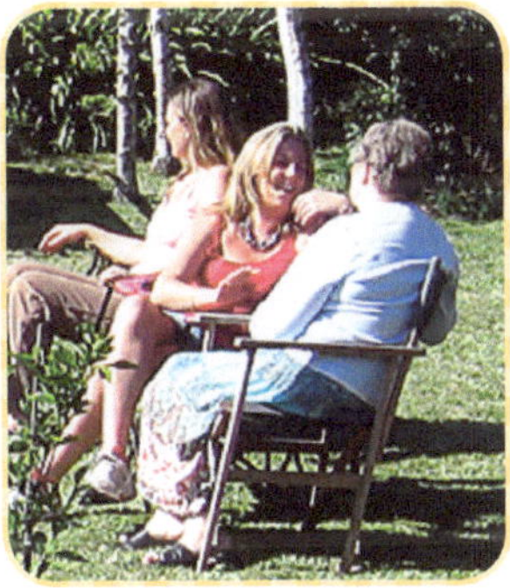

Your partner notices the three women sitting together, and recognises two of them as the local gossip clique. She notices how the two chatting are completely ignoring the third woman—probably making some bitchy comment about her clothes. She notices how the third woman has turned away, and decides that she will sit next to the poor girl. Your partner also notices how well the garden is kept. She notices the spread and thinks about the effort the hosts have gone to. The 'BEER' sign and Nugget's moon-salute escape her attention.

The reality is:

Kerrie and Mick are not having relationship dramas; Kerrie's just pissed off at her hubby for getting everyone else a drink but not her. Apart from that, they're one of the happiest couples you're likely to meet. The two ladies chatting together are not gossipping, they are deciding which one of them will go and tell the cook to hurry up, because they are starving. The third lady is not looking away because she's been spurned, she's looking over at her boyfriend, Nugget, who has dropped his strides, and she's thinking about what she can throw at him to stop him causing her further embarrassment. And yes, the hosts have gone to a lot of effort with the food. And yes, the garden is immaculate.

> ***Unique insight:*** Women are not crazy, emotion-charged, irrational creatures that were put on this earth to confuse and confound us men; they simply see the world differently to us. Once we accept this fact, then, and only then, will we find it much easier to cope with the wonderful mystery that is woman.

Chapter 8
She is not your mum

Remember what it was like when we were boys? Even though we tortured our sisters and the family pets, trashed our toys and generally caused mischief, we were still the apple of our mum's eye.

Do we remember all the work mum used to do around the house? Yes? We probably also remember that our aunties and grandmothers did the same. So it stands to reason that us blokes assume that we'll one day find someone to worship and care for us just like the female role models of our childhood did for their men.

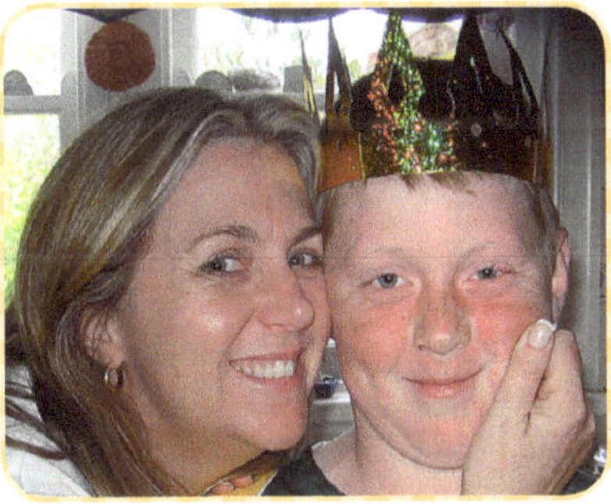

It's good to be King!

NEWSFLASH!
YOU'RE NO LONGER MUMMY'S LITTLE BOY,
AND TIMES HAVE CHANGED.

Nowadays, women have opportunities to forge careers for themselves. Becoming a housewife is a choice rather than a necessity. No longer is it taboo for a woman to be over 30 and single. If women are in the market for a partner, they want more than just a provider, and they definitely don't want someone to mother.

Key point: Think of women in terms of how they acted 30 years ago, or constantly compare them to your mother, and you'll be doomed to failure.

Chapter 9
What women really want from their men

Most men think they have some idea of what a woman wants from her man. A quick Q&A with the guys down at the pub revealed the following:

- A good provider.
- Someone who is respectful, trustful and sincere.
- A good father.
- A protector.
- Someone who is loyal.

When I asked those same guys how they came by their answers, most of them responded with: their mates, their dad, their uncles, their older brothers, films, books and magazines. Fellas, we don't have a clue what women really want, because we don't bother to ask them. And on the very rare occasions we do, we don't listen to the response, or we're so overwhelmed by the response that we ignore it and proceed to tell *them* what they really want. Allow me to shatter a few myths.

Not all women are looking for a hubby

That's right. Women are much more independent these days and can look after themselves. Sometimes they just want to have a bit of fun with us blokes, with no strings attached—whether that be clubbing, going to the movies or getting down and dirty with some stud-muffin whose name they'll never remember but whose body they'll never forget.

Some women are as shallow as men

Do us men honestly think that we're the only shallow ones on this planet? How do we explain the 'he's-a-bastard-but-I-still-want-to-shag-him' syndrome or the 'ugly-man-with-the-glamour-girlfriend' syndrome? The answer—some women couldn't give a hoot about the strength of our morals. They're more interested in traits such as:

- Physical appearance.
- Earning potential.
- Power.
- Fame.

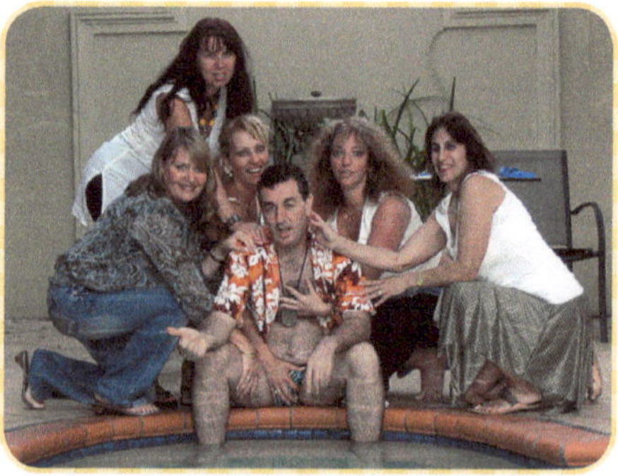

What has this bloke got that most of us haven't?

Women get bored

Just being a good father and provider is not enough these days. Women will get very bored, very quickly, with the same old routine. And when they do get bored, they begin to exercise their imagination; they begin to look for stimulation in chick-lit books and chick-flicks, searching for that sense of adventure and romance that we're not giving them.

For most women, imagination is where the fantasy ends, but if we're not careful, us blokes could find ourselves working our arses off to provide the best environment for our families only to watch helplessly as some hot-blooded Casanova—who looks like Antonio Banderas, makes love like a rampaging bull and drives a Ferrari—comes along and steals away the missus.

What do women want from their men?

Recently I spent the best part of a week asking women—single, married, divorced and those having affairs—the above question. What I got back was an absolute laundry list of wants and needs that included (in no particular order):

1. A man who makes me feel safe and secure.
2. A man who respects and supports freedom of choice concerning career and lifestyle.
3. A man who displays the fundamental core values of truth, honesty, sincerity, compassion, loyalty, generosity and respect.
4. A man who can make me laugh.
5. A man who's willing to share the domestic load.
6. A man who takes the time to pleasure me as well as receive pleasure.

7. A man who has a sense of adventure.
8. A man who inspires me.
9. A man who is passionate about life.
10. A man who looks after himself and spends a bit of time on grooming.
11. A man who knows when to take the lead and when to listen.
12. A man with rock-hard abs and who's hornier than a jack-rabbit.

The lucky few amongst us who are rich, famous, powerful or good-looking can pretty much ignore the above list and still find themselves with no shortage of babes to choose from. But for the rest of us, it is blatantly clear that women are demanding more of us than they ever have before. It's blindingly obvious that we can no longer sit on our arses and refuse to evolve if we hope to compete on the singles' scene or keep our long-term relationship happy and healthy. However, one look at the above list is enough to make most of us give up the ghost without even trying. I mean, who do these women think we are—Superman? But don't worry, help is on the way.

In the next part of the book I will unveil strategies that can transform even the ugliest no-hopers among us into charismatic love-machines capable of holding our own against any competition (including the rich, famous, powerful or good-looking blokes). The best thing about these strategies is that they don't require us to change too drastically, and getting the results won't require too much effort. Perfect!

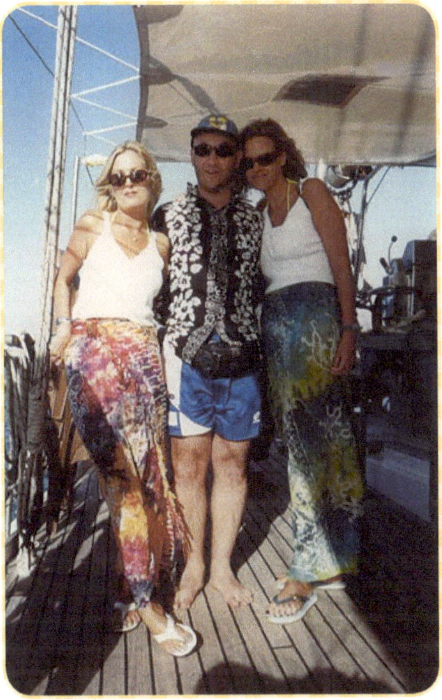

Even the ugliest no-hopers among us can hang out with beautiful ladies. If I can do it, so can you. Let me show you how.

Part 2 — Summary and conclusions

Being secure in our manhood is a vital first step in attaining happiness, but it won't help us understand the opposite sex. And if we're planning on finding ourselves a lady, or keeping the one that we have, then a better understanding of the womenfolk will go a long way to ensuring our success. Keep in mind the following key points:

1. Understanding everything there is to know about women is like herding cats—impossible! Us men should just accept the fact that women see the world differently and learn to go with the flow.
2. Under no circumstances should we expect our partner to be our mum.
3. These days, women want much more than just a good bloke who will look after them.

Us men must understand that we don't understand everything there is to understand about women, but the very understanding of this fact is the path to understanding—if you understand what I mean.
(Source: The book *Birds and Bees Speeches that Work*)

Our relationships with women — An introduction

The next three parts of this text examine the way us men conduct our relationships with the opposite sex. Before beginning this examination, it is important to note that our relationships with women follow a life cycle—a life cycle that involves our single days, followed by the commencement of a relationship, all the way through to a successful long-term relationship. I like to refer to this life cycle as the 'chasing the skirt' life cycle, and the way we travel through the life cycle goes a long way to determining our happiness. Please take a moment to examine the 'chasing the skirt' diagram on the next page before reading on. Pay special attention to the entry and exit points.

Parts 3, 4 and 5, which are to follow, are designed to equip us with the knowledge required to be successful in every phase of the life cycle; to enable us to smoothly journey through it while at the same time allowing us to get off at the exit point that will best ensure our happiness. This is instead of going round and round in circles, repeating the same mistakes over and over again until we eventually spin hopelessly out of control and end up so dizzy and confused that we jump off at an exit point we would rather avoid (nuts chopped off, early death or wearing the skirt). Are we ready for 'the knowledge'? We are? Then let's get into it.

From chasing the skirt to wearing one – the life cycle explained

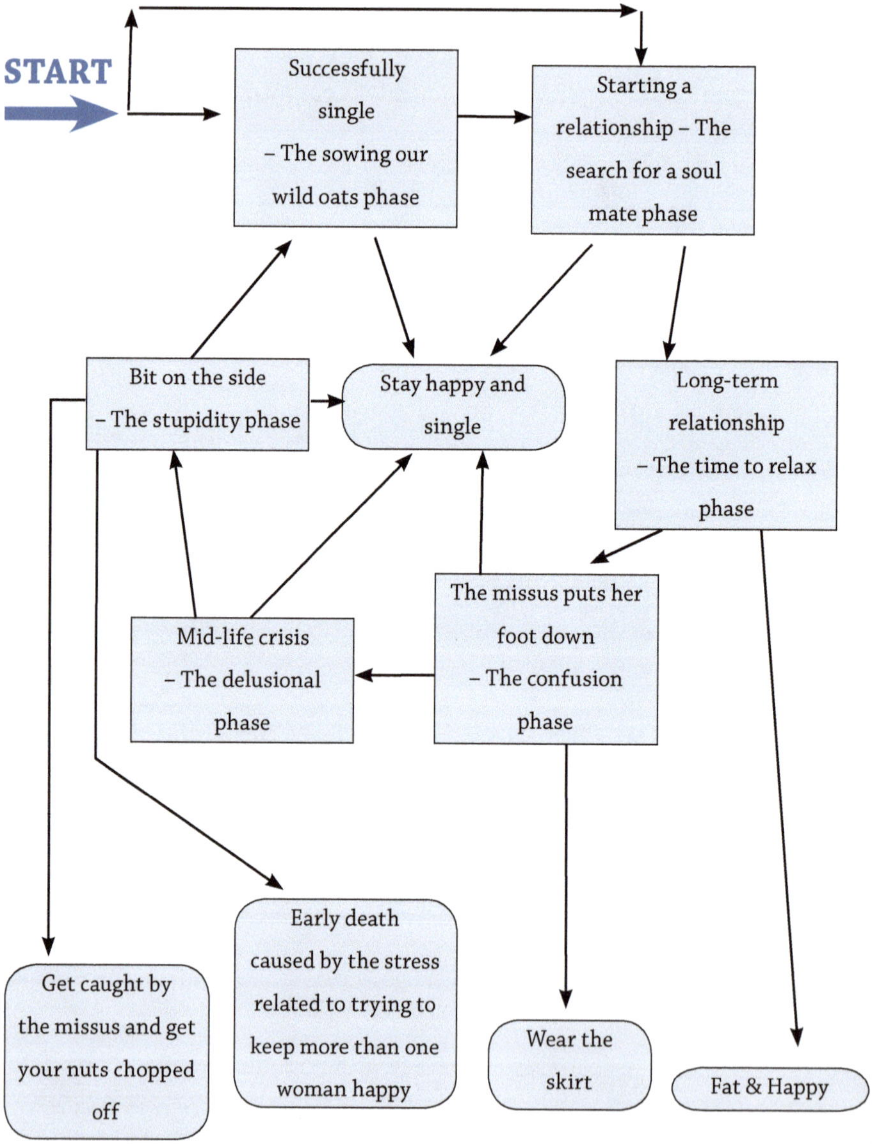

PART III

Successfully single

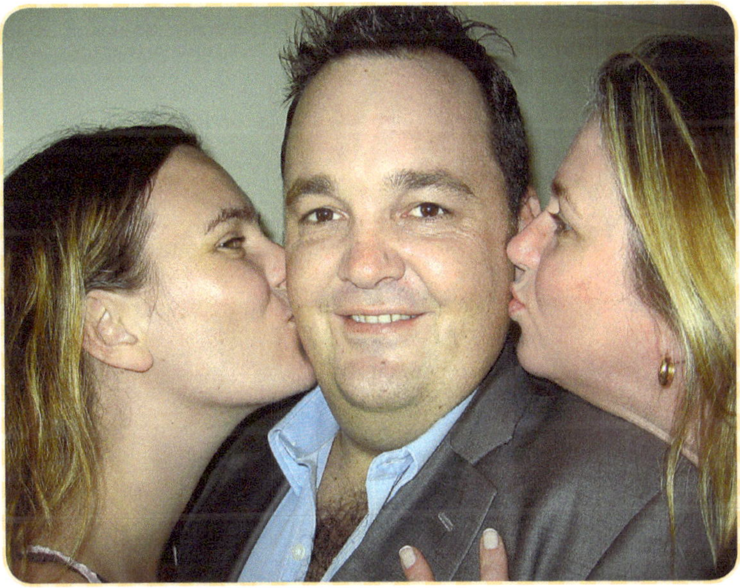

Chapter 10
Why are there so many unhappy singles out there?

In my capacity as a barman, I am staggered by the amount of single men that are unhappy with their lot. Being single should be a time of fun and mateship, of adventure and independence. It should be a time in our lives when we gather experiences and memories that we'll look back on fondly and recall with a smile when life throws its challenges our way; experiences and memories that we can use as bragging rights over all the other senior citizens when the kids have finally shipped us off to the nursing home.

When I dig a little deeper and ask these single men why they're so unhappy, I get a lot of responses that include reasons such as loneliness, emptiness, confusion, lack of direction and dwindling finances. Fellas, these are only surface symptoms of the root cause—a syndrome that I like to call 'bachelor burn-out'.

Bachelor burn-out

Many of us men have a vision of our single days as being one long sexfest. We picture ourselves moving from stunner to glamour to supermodel to doll to babe, racking up the notches in the belt as if it were as easy as shelling peas.

For most of us, though, the reality is a long way away from this vision. A more accurate description of our single days would be as a phase in our lives where we hit the nightspots and expend a lot of energy trying to pick up as many women as we can in an attempt to bang ourselves silly but more often than not come up empty-handed, eventually giving up the chase to hit the grog and pissing most of our money up against a urinal wall only to wake up the next morning in some strange place with a thumping hangover and an empty wallet, then proceeding to waste that whole day recovering in front of the computer with greasy takeaway in one hand while the other hand alleviates the frustrations of another night of no nooky, all the while racking up a monstrous Internet bill by giving the ol' broadband connection a thorough working over with downloaded erotica.

Knock-back after knock-back, hangover after hangover, will eventually lead to bachelor burn-out—a condition that overcomes us when expectations do not meet reality. To avoid it, we must learn to sow our wild oats successfully.

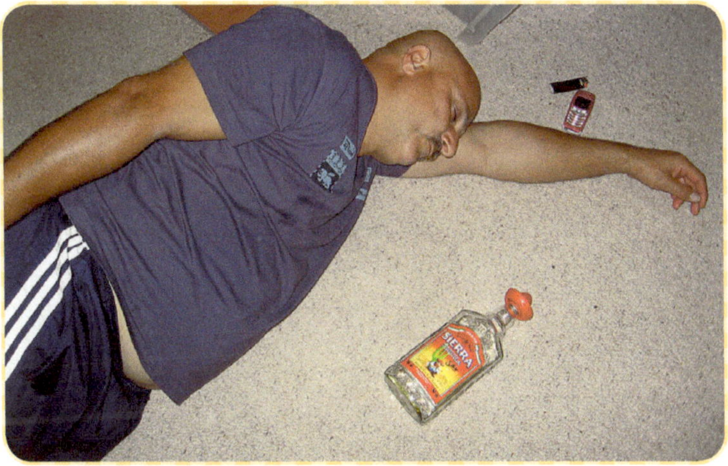

Bachelor burn-out.

Chapter 11
Sowing our wild oats successfully

Despite what us men have been conditioned to believe, sowing our wild oats is not just about acting like dogs on heat, trying to hump anything that moves. This type of behaviour can only lead to disappointment. To be successfully single, we need to adopt a more holistic approach. We need to understand that sowing our wild oats is all about taking the opportunity to use the freedom and independence of our single days to experience life to the full so we can be happily under the thumb later on in life.

Take the opportunity to travel

Most of the blokes I talk to regret not having taken the opportunity to travel. They had always intended to travel but for one reason or another they never got around to it. The main reason they never got around to it was that they got themselves into a long-term relationship, and then other factors such as starting a family or buying a house became more important than travelling. Sure, these blokes still hitch up the family wagon and head down to the trusty caravan park on the coast every Christmas, but they feel they've missed their opportunity to take that once-in-a-lifetime trip.

Before us blokes get too serious with a girl or settle into a career, we should all take some time out and go see the world, or at least our own country. Travel teaches us more about ourselves, and those around us, than anything we are taught at school. And the experiences and adventures that we enjoy during our travels will live in our memory for the rest of our lives. And when we do get the wife, the kids and the career, we'll enjoy them all the more because we'll have no regrets.

Travel tip: Try heading off the tourist track and spending as much time with the locals to maximise your cultural experience.

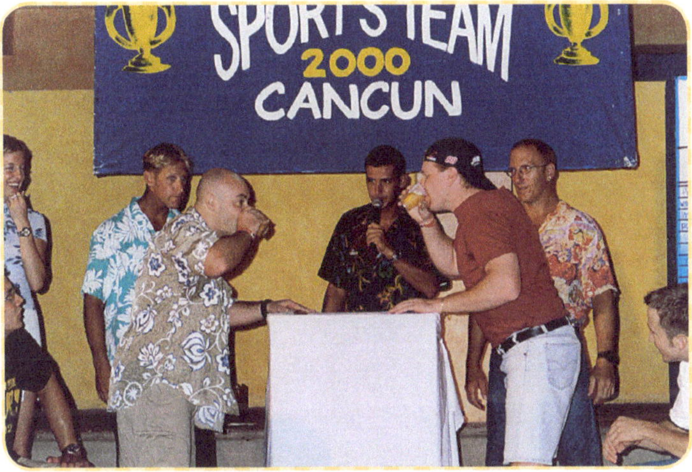

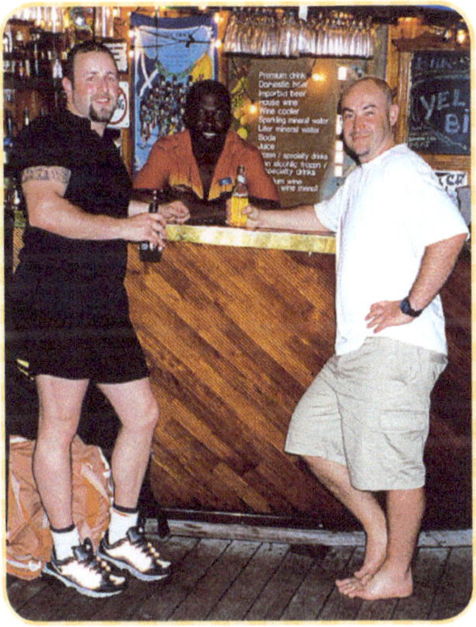

Happy snaps from the author's travels, including such varied and wonderful cultural experiences as representing his country in the Cancun International beer swilling race, and hangin' with the locals at the bar on a recent cricket lovers' tour of the West Indies.

Try as many different experiences as you can

When we're single, it's easy for us men to get into a routine of living for the weekends. We work hard each weekday, come home, watch a bit of TV and then collapse. The only thing that makes it all that bit easier is the knowledge that when Friday comes around, it's party time.

The problem is, when Friday does come around, most single men have got such a head-full of steam that they end up going nuts and getting lagered up in double-quick time. They then spend all Saturday recovering, only to do it all again on Saturday night; and before they know it, it's Monday again.

When we're single we should go out and experience as many different things as we can: white water rafting, opera, film festivals and so on. The more experiences we gain, the more rounded we become. And we shouldn't use money as an excuse, because there are plenty of experiences single blokes can have on the cheap—going bushwalking or nude parachuting are just a couple of examples. At the end of the day, we men don't want to get to 50 and think, *I wish I had tried that or done more of this when I was younger.*

Enjoying our mates

Once us men do get into a relationship, finding the opportunity to spend some quality time with our mates becomes increasingly difficult. And that's why we should make the most of the time we have with our mates when we're single. And this doesn't just mean getting lagered every weekend—it means card nights, going to watch some sport, gentlemen's clubs, porn and prawn nights.

Whatever we do, we should enjoy the time we spend with our buddies, because it won't last forever.

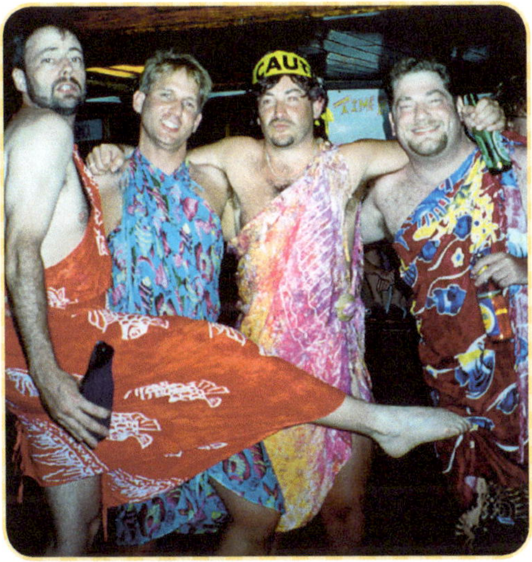

Mateship is a beautiful thing.

Don't see women as stats

Mixing with the fairer sex is an extremely important part of our single life, for this is the time when we learn the skills that will hopefully land us that 'special someone' we can spend the rest of our life with. Problem is, too many single guys out there have the wrong attitude, and end up learning nothing except the charms of Mrs Palmer and her five daughters.

There are lots of experiences we can have with the opposite sex that don't involve the 'wild thang'. Just spending time with them—on a date, on a trip away, at a dinner party—can be a rewarding and educational experience. All I'm saying is, don't start picturing them in lingerie at the first sniff of perfume; chill out and spend a bit of time getting to know them first—at least a few minutes.

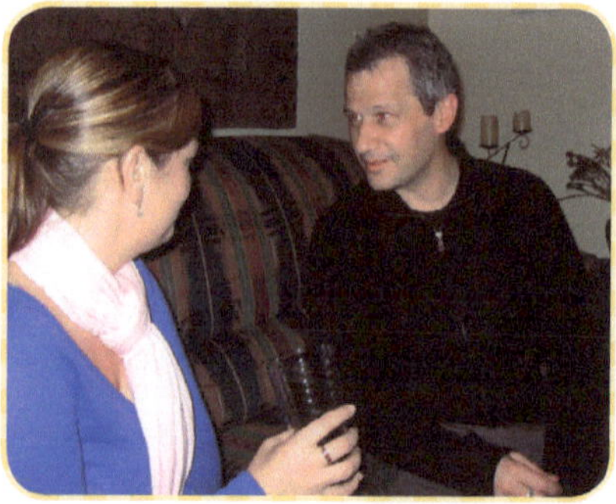

When conversing with the opposite sex,

instead of picturing her in these,

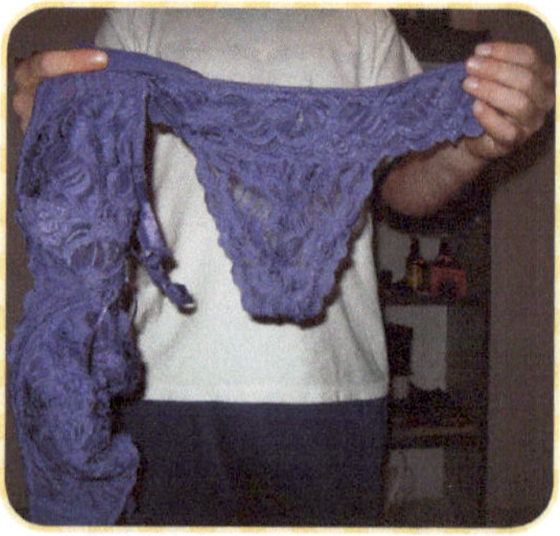

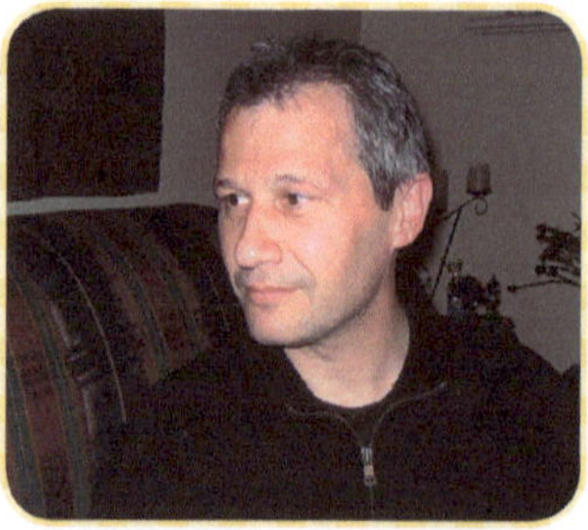

try keeping your mind on the conversation.

I know what you're saying: "WHAT'S THE POINT IN BEING SINGLE IF ALL I DO IS HANG OUT WITH MY MATES, TRAVEL, AND CHIT-CHAT WITH WOMEN? I WANT TO SCORE AS WELL." Okay, okay, I hear ya. But it's important we men understand that there's more to being single than just having sex. Having got that out of the way, now let me share some tips on how we can improve our chances of getting lucky!

Chapter 12
How to get lucky, even if you're ugly

Most single fellas find it difficult to get a bit of action because their attitude is all wrong. They believe that meeting women and spending time with them is their God-given right; that somehow, somewhere, some hot-looking chick who thinks the world of them will just fall out of the clouds, land in their laps and proceed to tickle their tonsils with her tongue. Keep dreaming, lads! You have to make it happen.

Doing our research, having a plan

If we're single and we're not rich, famous or good-looking, then 'getting lucky' is a numbers game. It's all about stacking the odds in our favour to improve our chances, and the way to do that is to do our research and have a plan.

Us men should think of our quest to meet women (and hopefully get lucky) in the same way we think about fishing. We wouldn't just rock up to a beach, cast in our worm and hope to catch a nice piece of trout. NO! We'd study the environment—the tides, the reefs. We'd take into consideration such factors as how many other fishermen are on the beach, whether anybody is catching anything, and if so, how? Is it too crowded? Should I find another spot? We'd think about the equipment we need to do the job—hooks, bait, lures and so on.

Successful fishermen do their research and have a plan. If we want to land ourselves a nice catch (instead of getting snagged in the weeds, catching nothing but an old shoe, or forever talking about the one that got away) then we need to do the same.

To save everyone time and energy, I have devised a '4-point-plan-to-landing-a-nice-catch' that we can all use; a plan that is easy to understand, simple to follow and guaranteed to stack the odds of getting lucky in our favour. Check it out.

The 4-point-plan

1. Understand your competition.
2. Put yourself where the girls are and the competition is not.
3. Advertise your wares.
4. Reel them in with your own X-factor.

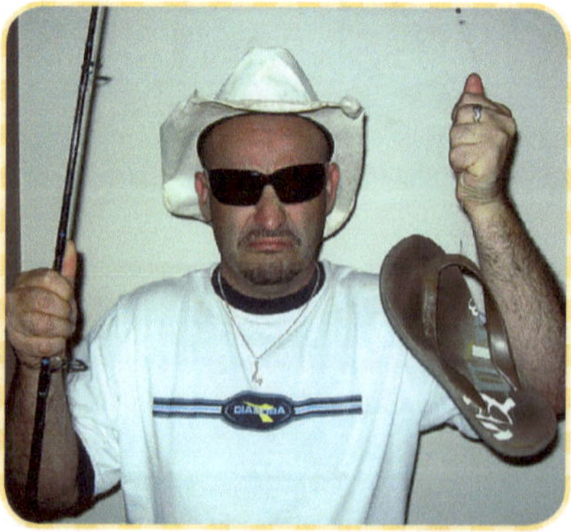

Sick of coming up with nothing but an old shoe? Use the 4-point-plan!

Chapter 13
Understanding our competition

There are four types of competitors that single men will encounter out there in the singles' jungle.

1. The NFI man

These guys fall into two categories:

a. 16-29 year olds. No strategy when it comes to getting laid. Clichéd chat-up lines are their only weapons besides alcohol (which they drink for courage and hope the ladies drink to excess). Usually give up on finding a lady, following one knock-back after the other, and just get hammered. Finish the night off singing old AC/DC or Chilli Peppers' songs arm-in-arm with their buddies and throwing up in a corner just before getting kicked out.

b. 30-80 year olds. Typically re-entering the singles' scene after experiencing a failed relationship, or seeking escape from a failing relationship. Usually suffering some sort of mid-life crisis and are hell-bent on recapturing their lost youth, or proving that they still 'have it'. This category is full of men who try to look half their age but just end up looking tragically desperate and old (ponytail being the hairdo of choice). Normally finish up wasted after a night out, with nothing to show for their endeavours. By midnight these guys have usually had enough and, consequently, retreat to a 'grab a granny night' at an over 35's nightspot, hoping for better luck in their own age group.

2. *The pants man*

This guy is your seasoned professional. Selective about the women he goes after (actresses, models or powerful female execs). Quality, not quantity, is his end goal. Always works alone, always has a plan. Usually possesses one of the following traits: good looks, wealth, fame, power or a huge schlong. Uses material possessions to his advantage—flash car, latest fashion accessories and so on. Can pick up the signs that a lady is interested very quickly, and uses stories of his achievements (whether they're true or not isn't important to him) to get her in the sack. This guy is the consummate talker, and his favourite subject is himself. What stamps him apart from the others is his ability to 'close the deal'. Once his mission is accomplished, this guy is an expert at the quick exit and cutting all ties, which allows him to move onto to his next conquest without complication.

3. The ladies man

Typically works alone, although can use a wing-man who he has trained to act uncouth in front of the ladies (a practice known as 'sending in the dog'). Generally has a rudimentary strategy that involves appealing to a lady's notion of 'the perfect gentleman'. Buys her drinks, pulls out her chair, opens her door and comments profusely on how beautiful she looks, or sends in the dog and then acts as the knight in shining armour by rescuing her. Most defining characteristic is his willingness to listen and empathise, even if in the back of his mind all he can think about is her in a bra and panties. Unlike the pants man, the ladies man has difficulty cutting ties—on account of his romantic methods—which typically results in women that want more than just a one-night stand. As a result, the ladies man usually ends up juggling more than one woman at a time—a situation fraught with danger.

4. The woodsman

These guys are the sharks of the singles' scene, and are single-minded in their intent. It's all about quantity. Not selective at all. Basically, they will try and mount anything that's not nailed down. They have no plan and no shame. Will not hesitate to butt in on another fella (a practice known as 'cutting someone else's grass') who is in the midst of chatting up a lady, and undoing all that fella's hard work with a direct, "Fancy a root?" Woodsmen work on the mathematical law of averages—the more women they proposition, the better their chances. These guys can cause chaos and are best to avoid at all costs.

Chapter 14
Location, location, location

"Location, location, location" should be the catchcry for real estate agents and single men alike. The best way to increase our odds of meeting women is to put ourselves where the women are and our competitors are not; and the only way to do that is to choose the right location.

Basically, places to meet women can be broken up into two categories: real world and the Internet. For now, I will concentrate on the real world, where locations such as pubs, clubs, gyms, workplaces, holiday destinations, singles-only dinners and speed-dating venues are the most well known of the 'pick-up' joints. The problem with these locations, however, is that they are usually full of other blokes trying to score, and too much competition is not what we want.

What do we want in a meeting place? We want locations where the man-to-woman ratio is low, where everyone shares a common interest so that we can easily start conversations with the opposite sex without having to resort to dodgy pick-up lines. Consider the following gems.

Top 5 Meeting Places in the 'Real World'

1. ***Join a dance club:*** Ballroom dancing is all the rage these days and by far the best way to meet women, because the odds are stacked in our favour. How? Dance clubs are usually full of women, with hardly a man in sight (most men still think of ballroom dancing as a pastime for pansies). We get to bump bits with lots of different women and we get fit in the process. Plus, when we do learn a few moves, we become more attractive to the ladies, because women can't resist a man that can dance.

I'd let a man touch my wife but never dance the tango with her.
(Source: A Spanish proverb)

2. ***Go swimming:*** One of the best-kept secrets of the modern age in terms of places to meet women. The local pool is full of ladies doing their laps and aqua aerobics, and all we need to do to get amongst it is pull on the Speedos and goggles and get wet.

   A swimming success story: My mate Dan met his wife at the local pool. He jumped into the fast lane and decided to do a fast lap. With goggles all foggy, he didn't notice the lovely lady 10 metres up the lane doing a slow breaststroke. He powered his way to mid-pool and, just as he was about to plough into her, she frog-kicked, resulting in him plunging nose first into her most private of parts. She yelped before slapping him; he was embarrassed and apologetic. A few minutes later they both laughed hysterically. They were married six months later and have been happy ever since.

3. ***Go to the races:*** Horse racing meetings are rapidly becoming the social events of the new millennium. The races are more about fashion these days than they are about horses, and they provide women with the ideal opportunity to frock-up and look glam—as well as an excuse to hit the champagne. So if we're looking to hook-up, we don the suit and shades, head to the races to study the form, and hopefully we back ourselves a winner.

4. ***Take a course:*** Adult learning centres are springing up everywhere. Courses such as pottery, lead lighting, painting and novel writing are full of women. But if we do enrol, then at the very least we choose a course that interests us, otherwise we run the risk of looking like fools.

5. ***Enlist in a cause:*** Women are nurturers by nature. They care about the world and are willing to get off their butts in order to help make it a better place. So while all the other single blokes are sleeping off hangovers, we get our butts out there and take part in 'Save the tree frog day' or 'Clean up Australia day'. Whatever the cause, we'll be surrounded by passionate women, plus we'll be doing our bit for the environment. Everyone's a winner.

Chapter 15
It's all about advertising

No doubt about it, for those of us that are single, choosing the right location is vitally important if we hope to improve our odds of partaking in a bit of hanky-panky. But even if we do find ourselves at a place where the odds are not in our favour, we can still compete—it's all about advertising.

Picture this: You walk into a party and it's chock to the rafters with single women. You've spent hours grooming yourself, donned the latest designer clothes, and you feel like you're in with a show. The problem is, there's a lot of other well-dressed, well-groomed men in attendance, and most of them are better looking than you. To add insult to injury, you suspect one or two of these well-groomed men are pants men plying their trade.

Most of us, when faced with the above scenario, would simply drop our head and resign ourself to playing second fiddle to all the pretty boys. But we don't need to. This is precisely the situation where us blokes should take a leaf out of Mother Nature's book. What do the males of many species use to attract their mate? They use colour, gimmickry and accessories. They puff themselves up, they show their plumage, they bellow their mating calls. The peacock is a classic example: it mesmerises the peahen with its colourful tail feathers. What do we in the human world have to rival the peacock's feathers in chick-pulling power— THE HAWAIIAN SHIRT!

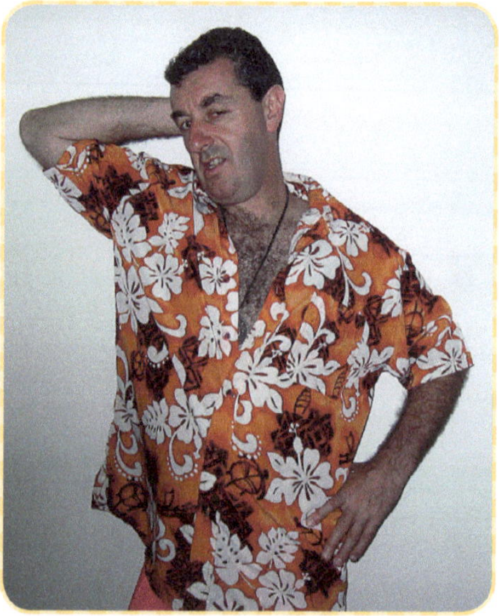

Never underestimate the power of the Hawaiian shirt.

The bottom line is, the best way for us to improve our chances with the ladies is to stand out from the crowd. We need to advertise. We need a way to make the women want to talk to us. And what better way is there than wearing a Hawaiian shirt? It's a winner!

If Hawaiian shirts are not our go

If, for some misguided reason, we're not comfortable wearing a Hawaiian shirt, then here are some other ways we can stand out from the crowd. Word of warning, though, WE DON'T OVERPLAY THE EFFECT! Subtlety is the key. We want the womenfolk to think us cute and endearing, not crazy nut-jobs that will do anything for attention.

Best ways to stand out from the crowd

1. We wear anything that glows, rotates or flashes.
2. We smoke tobacco out of an old-fashioned pipe, to give us an old-world charm, or a big-ass Cuban cigar for an aura of power.
3. We wear clothes that are way out of fashion (muscle shirts, tweed jackets, flared pants, cowboy boots). Because fashion goes in cycles, the ladies won't be too sure if we're at the forefront of a new look or have an account at the local opportunity shop—either way, they'll want to find out more.
4. We turn up in fancy dress, even though it's not a fancy dress party (superhero costumes are great). We wear lots of accessories: capes, wigs, ties—stuff that the ladies can take off of us, when they're smashed, and wear themselves. We're sure to be the talking point of the whole party.
5. We fake an injury. For example, we bandage a certain part of our body or we walk in on one crutch (if we do choose this option, we must be careful not to get too hammered and forget we're supposed to be injured).
6. When we venture out onto the dance floor—no matter

what music style is blaring through the speakers: dance, techno, jungle, garage, rock—we pick an animal and mimic its movements. My personal favourites are the 'praying mantis', for the slower tunes; the 'bounding gazelle' for the mosh pit; and the 'gorilla-gone-mad' works like a charm for frenzied techno.

7. We wear a kilt, no matter what nationality we are. Guaranteed, we'll have women lining up trying to work out whether we're 'real Scots'.

Chapter 16
Reeling them in

If we've advertised successfully, then sooner or later the womenfolk will come over and talk to us. The bad news is, once contact is made they will only give us one minute of their undivided attention. Therefore, we have a one-minute window of opportunity. One minute to make our sales pitch. One minute to wow their socks off. One minute to hook them or crash out in flames.

Common mistakes to avoid

Tacky chat-up lines

Most single men waste that one minute by using tired old chat-up lines in an attempt to 'break the ice'. More often than not, chat-up lines only serve to make the ladies cringe and automatically lose interest, so my advice is not to use them.

Top 5 'avoid-at-all-costs' chat-up lines

1. "Hey, somebody farted. Let's you and me get out of here."
2. "Would you like an Australian kiss? It's like a French kiss but down-under."
3. "Your parents must be retarded, coz you're S-P-E-C-I-A-L."
4. "Is that a Tic-Tac in your pocket or are you just glad to see me?"
5. "Do you have a band-aid? Because I just scraped my knee falling for you."

5 chat-up lines that 'reputedly' do the business

1. "You're so hot you'd make the devil sweat."
2. "Do you believe in love at first sight, or should I walk by again?"
3. "It's no use inheriting 80 million when I have a weak heart."
4. "Are those space pants you're wearing? Coz your ass is out of this world!"
5. "Fancy a chat? Don't worry, I won't try and chat you up. I promise!"

Do not be overpowered by 'The Horn'

The Horn

From the ages of about 12-14, men are afflicted with a powerful and potent force called 'The Horn'. The Horn has both a light and a dark side (the pants man is a prime example of the dark side of The Horn). When The Horn is at its most potent levels (during our teenage years), the mere whiff off a girl can shut our brains down completely and cause us great embarrassment. It can come on unexpectedly. Sometimes girls aren't even involved; something as innocuous as a gate opening and closing can bring it on. The power of The Horn may lessen as we age but it never really leaves us. Strange and mysterious is The Horn.

Just as animals can smell fear in the wild, women can sense the presence of The Horn—they can see it in our eyes. The Horn can make us men look and act desperate, so we must learn to control it. We must learn to subdue the beast in that critical first minute, otherwise it's game over.

Cursing, catchphrases, collective names and pranks

Cursing and catchphrases are a definite no-no. Nothing smacks of sleaze and piss-pot more than a few choice 'F' words. And catchphrases such as 'Who's ya daddy, baby', 'Keep it real', and 'Whazzup' simply make the ladies shut up shop. So too do collective names such as 'princess', 'duchess' or 'darling' (unless you're Jamie Oliver). And pranks such as the old 'butt-grab-whoops-thought-you-were-someone-else' routine are guaranteed to get you nowhere. Fellas, if we just talk normally we'll get a lot further in our conversations with the opposite sex.

How to reel them in successfully

If we do find ourselves at a party with the undivided attention of a lady, how do we best use our one minute to reel her in? We alter her reality.

The law of altered reality

A man's reality is visual, a woman's is visual and emotional. The trick for us men is to make women think and feel in such a way that they are not disappointed by what they see; to alter their sense of reality so they feel there is more to us than meets the eye. What we are talking about here is creating our own X-Factor.

Fellas, I ain't talking about spinning her a yarn about how we're marine biologists or jet fighter pilots. Women can see through that type of BS a mile away. What I'm proposing is much more complex, and requires practise, patience and skill. But the rewards are worth the effort. It's all about making a woman forget what she sees and concentrate on what she feels. How do we do this? We pique her curiosity, make her think there is more to us than meets the eye. Some men have heads like a beaten Melbourne Cup favourite, but the women still love them. Why? Because they have the X-factor—that mysterious quality that has the womenfolk yearning to find out more. We need to develop our own X-factor, and here's how to do it:

Creating our own X-Factor

1. **The passionate stare**
   We don't say a word in that critical first minute, we just stare into her eyes, trying to make it a stare that's brimming with passion. Passion has a killer effect on women; they can't resist a passionate man. They'll want to know what is fuelling that passion.

Tip for success: A method I like to use to get into the 'passionate zone' is to pretend I'm Rocky Balboa, standing toe-to-toe with Clubber Lang, with the Rocky theme playing in the background and the crowd chanting, "Rocky, Rocky".

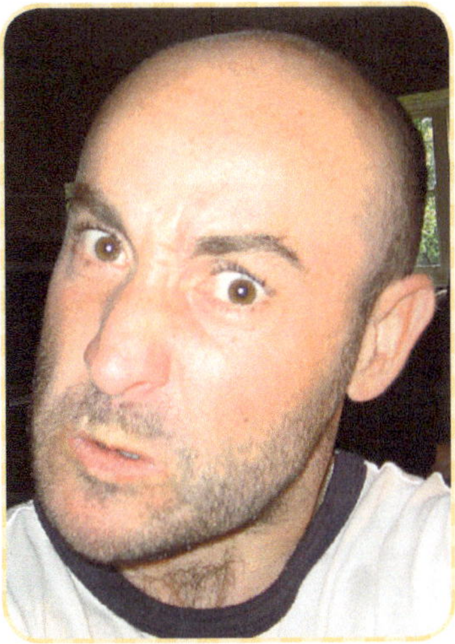

Passionate stares have a killer effect on the opposite sex. The photo above is of the author entering the 'passionate zone'. And the photo below is his partner's response. She is obviously impressed.

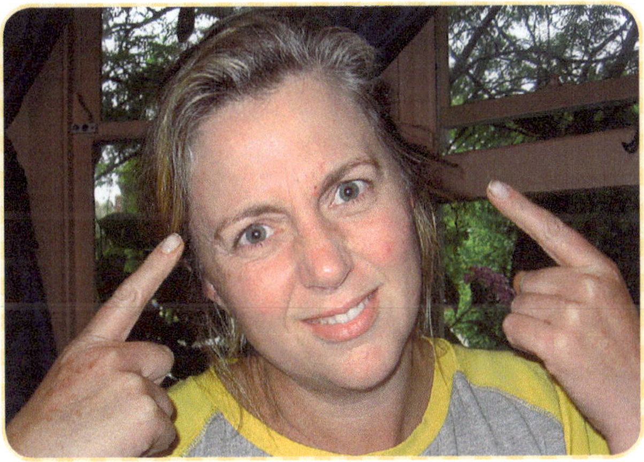

2. **Shed a tear**

   Tearing-up is another potent method for generating curiosity, but it does take a lot of practise. Again, we don't say a word in that first minute. We tear-up, timing it so the tear runs down our cheek at the 50-second mark. We make sure she sees the tear, and then we turn and walk away. Guaranteed, she'll want to know what has made us so sad, and when she does catch up with us again, we smile warmly at her and apologise, explaining to her it was a tear of joy. She will be intrigued.

Tip for success: If you find it difficult to tear-up on demand, then carry a freshly cut onion in your handkerchief. When it comes time to shed a tear, just whip out the hankie and blow your nose. Easy-peasy!

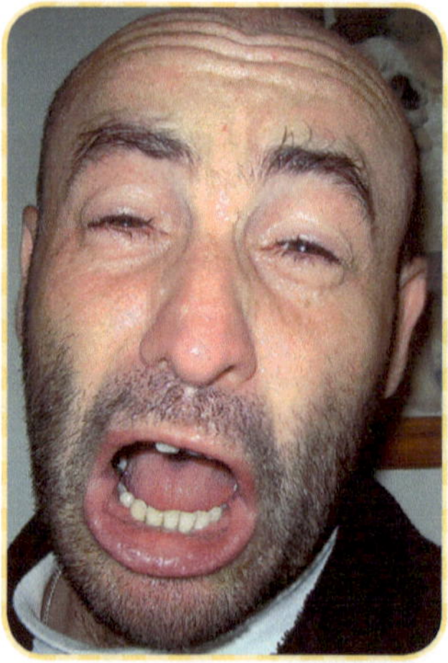

When utilising the 'shed a tear' technique, make sure your eyes are nice and moist and you adopt the facial expression designed to make maximum impact.

3. Make her feel sorry for you

Playing the sympathy card is another sure-fire way to get her wanting to know more. There's a couple of ways to do this.

a. Little-boy-lost routine. We look disorientated. We tell her we don't really know anyone at the party and we're glad we have someone to talk with.

b. We get a few mates to come along and poke fun at us while we're talking to her. And after the mates are finished with their taunts and jibes, we turn to her with our most sad and pathetic face before looking down at our shoes.

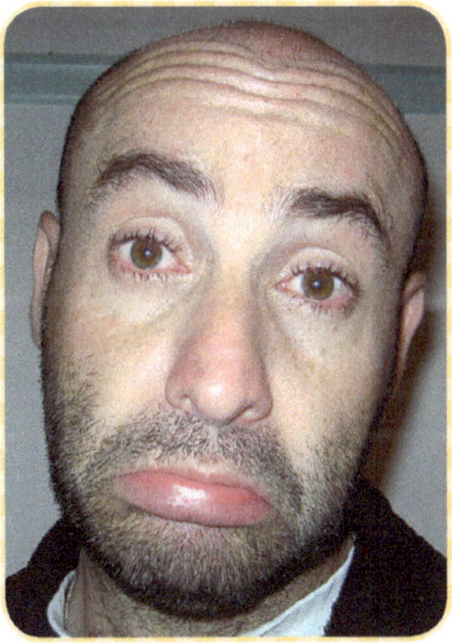

The little boy lost — a winner with the women.

4. **Sing her a song in a foreign language**
   As soon as we have her undivided attention, we burst out into song—singing in a foreign language. She will think us spontaneous and cultured, and she'll be putty in our hands (unless we're unlucky enough to pick out a girl who speaks the language we're singing in and thinks we're dickheads for mispronouncing all the words).

Tip for success: For greater effect, try combining the passionate stare, shedding a tear and bursting out into song. Use a guitar if you have one handy.

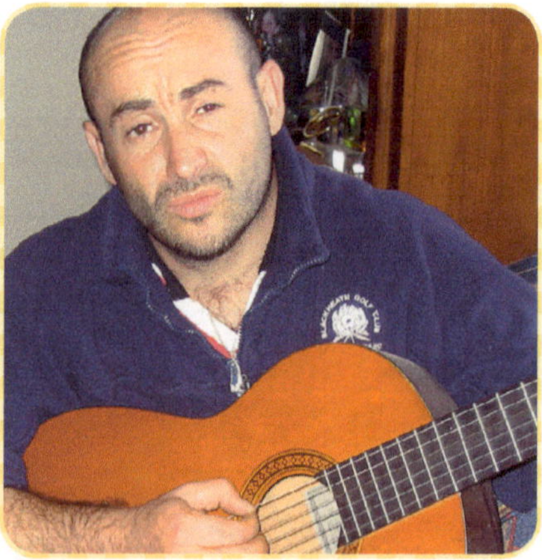

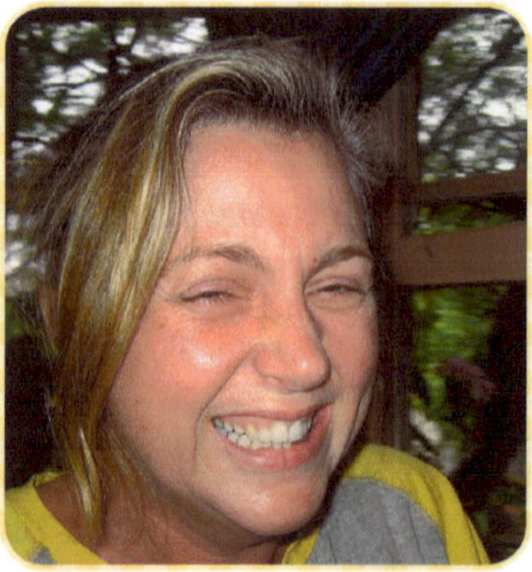

Nothing gets a gal going like a man singing and strumming his guitar. Just take a look at the author's partner, who is obviously overwhelmed.

5. **Smile**
   Human beings are attracted to other human beings who exude warmth and happiness. Next time we meet a lady for the first time, don't say anything and just smile at her for that critical first minute. She'll keep asking what we're smiling about, and each time she does we just smile even wider. Either she'll think we're a nut-case or she'll be smiling back, thinking what a beautiful spirit we have. She'll also want to know what's making us so happy.

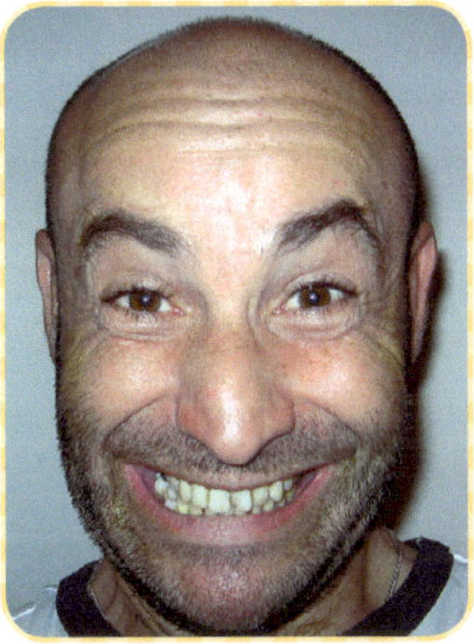

Why use words to win a heart when a winning smile will do?

In summary

We don't have to be an Adonis to meet women, we just have to have a certain way about us that piques their curiosity and leaves them wanting to get to know us better (the X-factor). Keep in mind, when meeting a lady for the first time, the first minute is critical and we must use it wisely. But even if the lady walks away after that first minute, we don't panic (on the singles' circuit, women rarely stop at the first guy they meet; they like to window shop, check out their options), because if we've used our one minute wisely, then sure as sheep shite on a shearer's shorts, she'll be back later for a second look (or sooner if she's got no better options).

One more thing, there are enough arseholes out there on the singles' scene without us joining their ranks. So when dealing with the opposite sex, we conduct ourselves with a bit of class

A code of conduct for the single gent

- Be honest. If a casual relationship is all you're after, then tell her before it all gets too hot and sweaty. In times past, telling a woman that you're there for a good time and not a long time would probably result in a slap on the mouche, but these days women are much more adventurous, and she may be looking for the same thing. If that's the case, you've hit the jackpot, sonny—Ka-ching!
- Always be respectful.
- Learn to take a "no" with good grace. If, after a while, she realises that she's no longer interested, or she spots a better option, take it on the chin and move on.
- Learn to say "no" with good grace. If you realise you're really not that interested, or you've spotted a better alternative, then let her down gently. Never burn your bridges—she may have a really hot friend.

Chapter 17
Internet dating success

Now that we've dealt with meeting women in the real world, let us turn our attention to cyberspace. A word of warning, though: us blokes should steer clear of the Internet if all we're after is a casual relationship. Why? Because the Internet is home to more freaks than a Star Trek convention, and if we're not careful we could end up at a swingers' party full of hairy-backed Neanderthals waiting to dress us up in a gimp outfit and ride us like a pony.

On the other hand, if we have the social skills of Hannibal Lecter or look like Ozzy Osborne, then the Internet does have certain advantages over the real world singles' venues:

- No sleazy, smoke-filled singles' bars to navigate.
- It's a relatively cheap way to meet the ladies.
- There are literally thousands of Internet dating sites with thousands of members, so there is no shortage of ladies to choose from.

- You can be ugly as sin and still have a chance of hooking up.

So how do we find a lady-friend on the Net? We use the same fundamentals we would in the real world—we understand our competition, we choose the right location and we advertise in a way that makes us stand out from the cyber-crowd.

Competition

Nothing is what it seems on the Net. Internet dating sites are rife with bogus profiles of men who are overselling themselves in order to get a step ahead. There is nothing stopping a scrawny, 5 foot 5 inch geek posting a picture of himself as a 6 foot 6 inch Mr Universe entrant who is so well-muscled he looks like a condom stuffed with walnuts. So how do we compete? How do we stand out in a world full of men who are overselling themselves? The answer—we undersell ourselves and we target a niche audience. Confused? Stick with me.

The Ben Stiller effect

Yes, Ben Stiller—the perfect role model for underselling. The star of such films as *Meet the Parents*, *There's Something about Mary*, *Dodgeball* and *Starsky and Hutch*. A guy who can poke fun at himself, who doesn't take himself too seriously, who is sensitive and can make the girls laugh; a guy whose quirkiness inspires affection.

I mean, let's be honest, Ben is nothing special in the looks department, but find me a girl who doesn't think he's genuinely a great guy. And in an Internet world full of fakes, women respond to genuine. So when we do come to posting our profile on a dating site, we should poke a bit of fun at ourselves, try a bit of humour, throw a few curve balls of quirkiness into the mix and show a bit of sensitivity.

Target a niche audience

Most men advertising themselves on the Net compile their profiles in a way that is designed to appeal to a mass audience, in the hope of increasing their chances of getting a reply. They load their profiles with generalised statements: love going to the movies, love going for walks on the beach, am a romantic at heart and so on. Bad move. In the business world, companies don't try and sell their products to everyone, they target their audience. When posting our profiles on the Net, we must do the same.

How do we go about it? We put hobbies and interests in our profiles that are specific to certain interest groups—the more niche the better. Why? Because people in niche groups like to stick together, and because of that, the chances of us getting a reply increase. Groups such as country music lovers, the Ewok fan club or the Nude Sailing Association. But we stay away from fetish groups, unless we want some leather-clad, whip-brandishing dominatrix knocking at our door looking for her new man-bitch.

Allow me to demonstrate the use of the 'Ben Stiller effect' and 'targeting a niche audience' by showing you a profile I set up recently on **www.aussiedesperados.com**

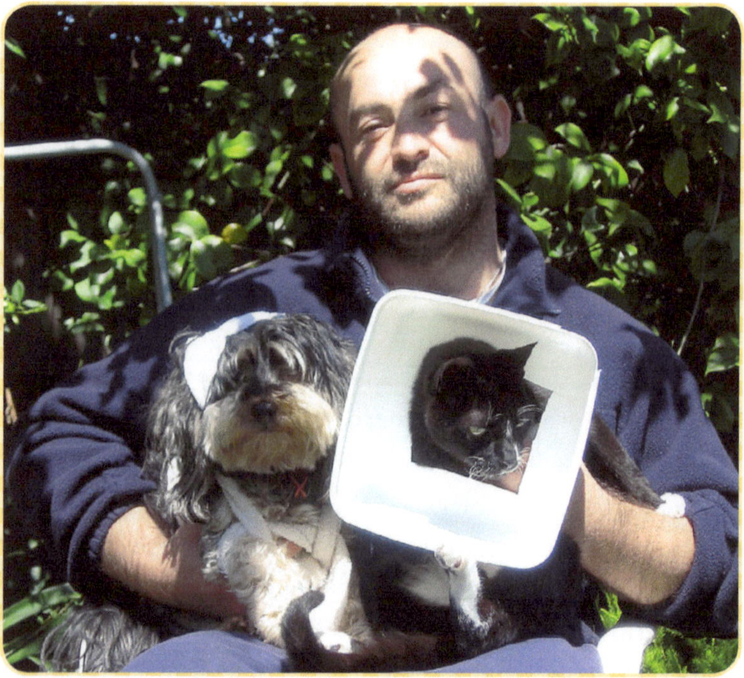

Member Name: Dr Luurv.

Age: Thirties.

Body type: Needs improvement.

Hair Colour: Brown with a bald spot on top as a result of one too many u-turns under the doona

Eye Colour: Bloodshot-blue.

Smoker: Yes, Cubans.

Drinker: Yes, vodka straight out of the bottle, Boris Yeltsin style.

Status: Single.

Children: Only my pets: my dog Doofus and my cat Shagger.

Religion: Jedi.

Occupation: Would love to work in a zoo.

Sign: Pisces.

Aim in life: To be happy.

Interests: Documentaries about animals.
Ideal partner: An animal lover who loves like an animal and wants to be loved by an animal.

Beautiful piece of work, isn't it? I've shown a quirky side that makes me seem genuine and interesting. I've also cornered the 'animal-lovers' audience by taking my profile photo in a wilderness setting and remaining bearded-up, Grizzly Adam's style. I've also shown my sensitive side by holding onto a couple of pets that look like they've met with the wrong end of a moving vehicle. Every Cathy-cat-lover and Dorothy-dog-owner will be falling over themselves to send me an e-mail of introduction. Mission accomplished.

Golden rules for Internet dating

Once we've posted our profile on the Net, we must keep in mind the following golden rules if we want our Internet experience to be a good one:

1. Don't be fooled by profile pictures. A stunning looking lady in a latex nurse's uniform who loves sex day and night and is willing to serve us beer while we flick from one sports channel to another on the TV *DOES NOT EXIST!*
2. Don't hand over credit card details or cash. Women we meet on the Net that ask us for money are phoneys. Simple as that.
3. Stay local. Those of us looking for love on the Net should limit our e-mail relationships to ladies that live in our local area, otherwise we could end up forking out a small fortune on airline tickets and hotel rooms.

4. We keep our clothes on. All of us should be extra careful if indulging in some kinky cyber-sex—especially if there's a web-cam involved. Anything we do on the Net that involves voice or image recording can be used against us by unscrupulous operators. The last thing we want is an e-mail containing a video of us parading around the bedroom in nothing but a Zorro mask and a pair of Speedos, sensually massaging ourself with oil while Ravel's *Bolero* plays in the background, being posted to the four corners of the globe.

The golden rule of golden rules

5. Don't fall in 'e-love'. E-love is where two people meet on the Net, exchange e-mails for months, or even years (commonly called an 'e-relationship'), and fall in love with the e-mail persona but not the actual person. Fellas, WE CANNOT TRULY FALL IN LOVE WITH SOMEONE WE HAVEN'T MET FACE-TO-FACE. If we find ourselves in an e-relationship and we think we really dig the person on the other end of the cable, then we arrange to meet her face-to-face as quickly as possible, and spend some time with her in the real world before deciding whether we want to pursue the relationship further.

So get online and have fun, but remember the old warning—buyer beware!

Chapter 18
A single man's guide to sex

Young and single

Taking the time to think about sexual technique is almost impossible for a young single bloke. It is a time in our life when we are so overcome by The Horn that our bodies behave in ways that seem beyond our control. During this time, most of us feel like our penis has a mind of its own and if we don't stick it somewhere or give it some 'self luvin' it will explode on us. It is a very delicate period, where merely the first rays of sunshine filtering through the bedroom window are enough to bring on a boner strong enough to break a woodpecker's beak (a phenomenon known as 'morning glory').

No doubt about it, when we're young and single we're at our prime in terms of desire and sexual energy. So much so that we're capable of superhuman feats, like walking around the house 24-7 with a towel hanging off of our old fella, just to impress our mates, the ladies or ourselves. On the flip side, however, if we do get a shot at a bit of nooky, we get so excited that we go about it as if we were wrestling in the Olympic Games, attempting to throw our bed-pal into all kinds of different positions in the space of a minute, none of which are practical and nearly all uncomfortable, only to finish up early, leaving her frustrated and thinking, *What an amateur.*

Mature and single

The more mature singles amongst us are likely to encounter a different type of problem when it comes to sexual technique—the 'sexual knowledge gap'. For a lot of the more mature gents, for one reason or another, it's probably been a while since they saddled up and went for a ride. So when the opportunity does arise, they go about it like they did many moons ago, only to discover that their lady-friends are no longer willing to lay back and think of England. All of which makes the mature single feel extremely incompetent (especially if their lady-friend begins giving them hints and directions).

Sure, when we're single, young or old, there are times when most of us blokes just want to get our rocks off; when we don't want to put on a song and dance; when we couldn't give a brass razoo what our bed-pals think or feel. But if we take a bit of pride in our work, if we want the ladies to think, *Now there's a man who doesn't need a map to send me to heaven*, then the following advice will prove indispensable.

Research

We should never trust what our mates tell us about sex. Many men tell 'tall stories' just to hide the fact that they know bugger-all. I'm sure we've all been on the wrong end of a myth or some bad advice. When I was 18 I was told by a friend that spitting in a girl's ear would turn her on, and I believed him. Why? Because he'd read it in a men's magazine; so he was an expert on the matter and who was I to argue?

And we should not assume that knowledge about sex is instinctive, that when the time comes us men will know where everything goes and how it all works. The best course of action, in case we get some action, is to be prepared—and the best way to prepare is with research.

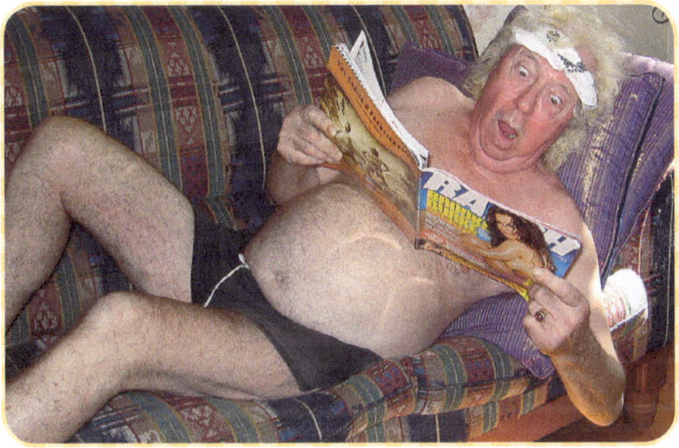

Next-door-neighbour Dave getting in some much-valued research, proving you're never too old to learn.

Research tips

There is an incredible amount of literature devoted to modern sexual practices, written by both men and women. Classics like the *Karma Sutra* are readily available. My advice would be to concentrate on articles prepared by females, as they know best what gets their motor running.

Handy hint: Next time you're in a waiting room, pick up a copy of *Cosmo* or *Cleo* and take a peak at the sealed section. This may strike you as dodgy behaviour but it's actually research. Guaranteed, you'll be staggered by how much you don't know and how much you can learn. Alternatively, hit the Internet and Google 'female erogenous zones map'. Trust me, you'll be gobsmacked by what you discover.

Discovering a woman's sexuality is like discovering Wonka's chocolate factory—a world you never knew existed, a world full of things you never thought possible; and best of all, you can taste and lick almost everything.
(Source: Unknown)

Practise

Mastery of sexual techniques only comes with experience. But when we're single (even though we may brag about the quantity of our sexual conquests—especially after a few beers) the chances of getting some much-needed experience are typically few and far between. The only way to short-circuit this sexual catch-22 is to practise by ourselves.

Tip for success: Rent yourself a couple of adult flicks from your local video library and take note of how the professionals go about their work. Pay special attention to their stance and positioning. Try practising what you see.

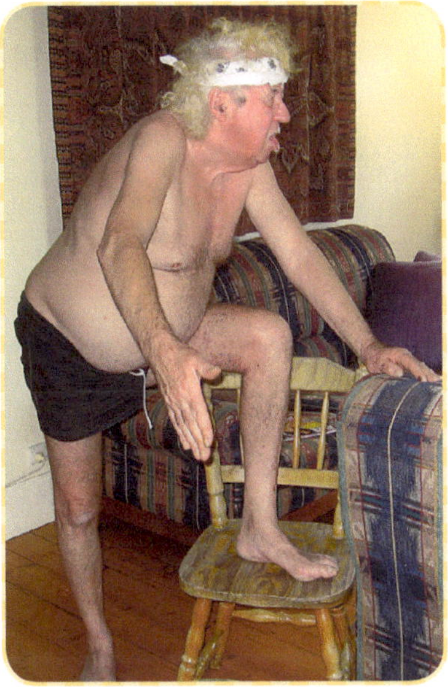

Dave practising the 'booty slap' position discovered while conducting research.

The four 'E's' of sex-cess

1. **Elasticity**

   So we've done our research and practised our technique, and gods be good, we've actually found a lady who's willing to do the wild thang with us. One of the main mistakes single men can make at this juncture is to dive in head first without preparation. If we're a little on the portly side, or we're not the fittest bloke in the world, then we're liable to do ourselves a serious injury unless we do our stretches. Stretching will help avoid soft tissue injuries like 'coitus-groin', 'doggy-style-disc-slip' or 'cunnilingus-neck'. Another advantage of doing our stretches is it will give us some time to calm ourselves so it's not all over before she's even had a chance to break a sweat.

2. **Excitation**

   Us blokes tend to get excited at the drop of a hat—especially if we're in the midst of a sexual drought—and most of the time we're ready to go before our pants have even hit the carpet. Our primal instincts make us want to go straight for the honey-pot and start whacking away like there's no tomorrow. We may get our enjoyment, but do our bed-pals? Single men who take the time out to help arouse their bed-pals are looked upon with much more respect by the womenfolk out there than men who don't. Foreplay is the term for it, and nowadays it involves a good deal of tongue work, which can be daunting for the inexperienced amongst us, especially when that tongue work is required below the high tide mark (if you get my drift). If you're worried about going 'down under' and making a fool of yourself, then the following may help.

Handy hint: Make a bowl of jelly (jell-O for our American friends) and drop an olive into it before it sets. When it has set, bury your head in the bowl and try to get that little sucker out using just your tongue. Next time you're with your woman, she'll be giving your ears a real good wrenching as you do your thing. And when you finish up, she'll be well satisfied and likely to look dreamily into your eyes and say, "Luv your work, baby." It'll be like all her Christmases have come at once. Soo-perb!

For those of us not into tongue work, there are other ways we can get our bed-pals going: sensual massage, stroking, nibbling, even the simple kiss can be a powerful turn on. If we're unsure, we shouldn't be afraid to ask our bed-pals for advice on what works for them. The point is, if we take the time to help our bed-pals get aroused, then even if we're hopeless at it, we'll be a much better option in their eyes than the bloke who just pleases himself.

Another handy hint: Women like us to undress them during foreplay, but nothing smacks of amateurism like a man who rips and pulls at bra-straps or suspender-clips because he's got no idea how to get the buggers off. But are us men ever taught how to undo a bra-strap? It's not like our fathers take us aside and say, "Son, you're a grown man now, so today I'm going to teach you how to shave and undo a bra strap." Teach yourself. Be proactive. Get yourself down to the local lingerie shop, buy yourself some gear and then practise, practise, practise. Next time you need to do a bit of undressing you'll be as cool and precise as a bomb squad technician, and she'll know she's dealing with a pro.

3. **Execution**

   Too many single men try to do too much when it comes to 'making love'. Just because they've seen Brad Pitt or Tom Cruise jumping off beds, bouncing off walls or hanging upside-down while going at it with their on-screen lovers don't mean that we can do the same—those guys have stunt doubles. A far better option for most of us, when it comes to executing sexual technique, would be to adopt the KISS principle (Keep It Simple, Stupid)—especially if we're caught in a confined space, such as an elevator, the back of the car or an abandoned garbage dumpster. We should pick a few positions and a few techniques and learn to do them well. If we try to do too much too quickly, we'll end up worrying more about our style and less about enjoying the moment, and our bed-pals will get sick of being flipped, twisted or rolled as if they were giant pancakes.

4. **Endurance**

Always a tough issue for us men. Most of us would like to be known as 'stayers' rather than 'sprinters', but how do we improve our endurance? Some men picture revolting scenarios in their mind, others count sheep. There are many different methods out there, but by far the most successful in my opinion is for us men to pick a piece of music to hum in our head while making love.

Tip for success: Pick a piece of music that goes for a while and has periods of both slow, and up-tempo, with maybe a guitar riff or two (but steer clear of music that is continuously up-tempo, like 'Turning Japanese' or 'The William Tell Overture', unless you want to make love like a battery-powered toy gone haywire). Any songs from the rock group Queen work well, as do 'The 1812 Overture' and 'Zorba the Greek'. As you begin your lovemaking, hum the tune in your head and match your tempo to the beat. Be careful not to blurt out parts of the tune or sing parts of the song out loud, otherwise you may find yourself having to explain to your partner why you're belting out the chorus to 'Bohemian Rhapsody' in the throes of ecstasy instead of calling out her name.

In summary

A good tradesman—be he electrician, plumber or mechanic—keeps up to date with the latest developments in his trade, including industry best practice and technological advances. He takes pride in his work, and if he does a good job at keeping his customers happy then not only does he get repeat business, he also gets referrals. Us blokes should do the same if we want to become 'Master Tradesman of the Shag' rather than just some clumsy apprentice.

Part 3 — Summary and conclusions

Most of us have at least one mate who's absolutely hopeless on the singles' scene. If we ask these hopeless cases why they're so hopeless, we're guaranteed to hear the same old excuses over and over again—I'm not good-looking enough; I'm not rich or famous, powerful or talented. Excuses, excuses, excuses. The truth is, us blokes don't need to look like a movie star or have a wallet as fat as a media tycoon's to pull the chicks. If we follow the 4-point-plan-to-landing-a-nice-catch then we'll be up to our armpits in gorgeous babes. If my mate Joey M (pictured overleaf) can do it (and trust me, he's no oil painting) then so can you.

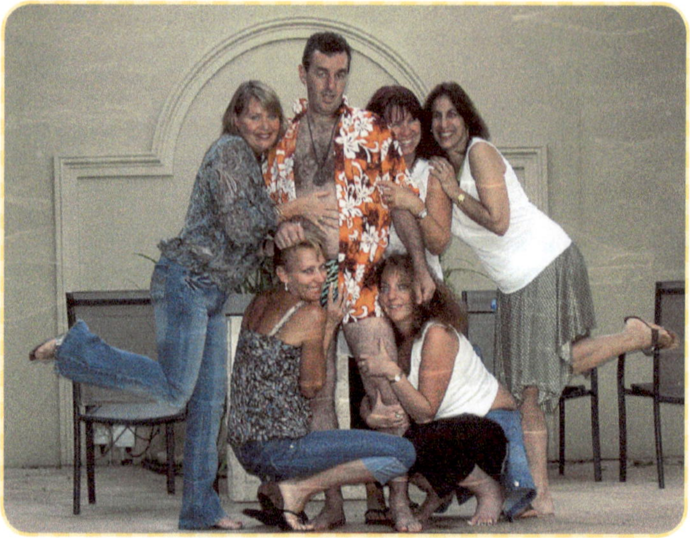

PART IV

Starting a relationship

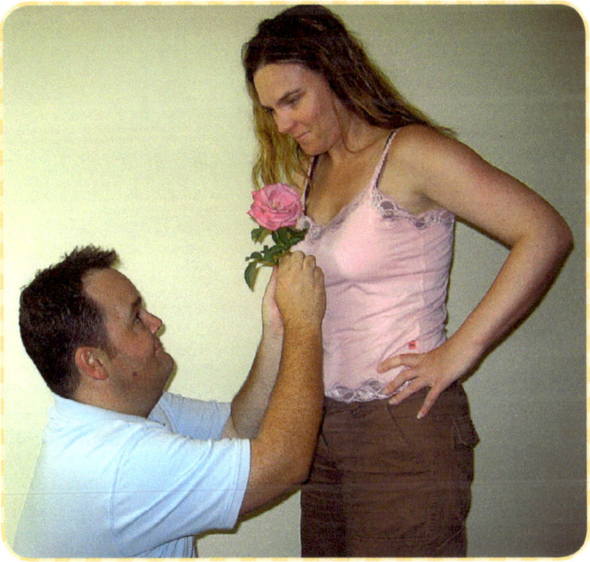

Chapter 19
Am I ready for a steady girlfriend?

Gentlemen, there's a big leap from being in a casual relationship to being in a steady relationship. Before us men jump headfirst into getting ourselves a steady girlfriend, we should ask ourselves, "Am I ready?" We should also examine our motives.

The wrong reasons to get yourself 'birded-up'

1. Time to give the liver and the wallet a rest

Most of us, at some point in our bachelor days, will suffer from bachelor burn-out (a period when we get sick of the singles' circuit and look for ways to give our livers and our wallets a rest). Getting ourselves a girlfriend seems to be the perfect solution, or is it? Bachelor burn–out is only a temporary affliction, and a week or two's respite from our mates is usually enough to have us well rested and ready to get back on that party horse with all guns blazing. But if we've gone and gotten ourselves a girlfriend before we've had a chance to get over our burn-out, then we may find ourselves feeling like trapped tigers when we're ready to start partying again.

The moral of the story is: we should never get ourselves a steady gal just because we need a break from the lads, otherwise we may find ourselves getting into a relationship before we have successfully sown our wild oats; and not successfully sowing our wild oats will come back and bite us on the arse later on in life. None of us want to be that middle-aged bloke sitting at the bus stop leering over the top of his newspaper at all the pretty young things sauntering past. Or the old geezer in the nightclub pinching the girlies on the bum, and in return copping a few slaps across the chops and the occasional "Keep your hands to yourself, you old pervert" for his troubles.

Lesson learnt: If necessity is the mother of all invention, then not making the most of your bachelor days is the mother of the mid-life-crisis.

2. All my mates are hooked up

When we're single, us blokes typically hang out in groups, and as soon as one or two of the group get hooked up then the others drop like nine-pins, until the last one in the group has no choice but to get himself a girlfriend or risk becoming the perennial 'third wheel'. Fellas, before starting a relationship we must learn to ask ourselves, "Is it my mates I'm missing or am I truly ready for the joys of a relationship?" If it's our mates, then we need to find more mates and stay single, because we're not ready for a girlfriend.

3. The potential for regular sex

The concept of sex-on-tap is as elusive, mysterious and ultimately unattainable as the idea of the fabled 'fountain of youth'. However, just as it is with the mythical fountain, so it is with sex-on-tap—everyone wants a piece of it. We could always pay and get sex-on-tap, but very few of us have that kind of coin and there are health risks involved. Or we could aim at getting ourselves one of those extremely rare creatures known as a 'sex-buddy'; but let's face it, our chances of hooking up with a woman who's up for sex day and night with no strings attached are similar to our chances of winning the lottery. Given that sex-on-tap is a myth and sex-buddies are as rare as hen's teeth, how do most blokes figure they're going to get themselves some regular booty? By getting birded-up.

Lads, listen up—if the only reason for getting ourselves a girlfriend is the idea that we'll no longer have to put in the hard yards to get ourselves some nooky, then we should think again and stay single, because there's a lot more to relationships than just sex.

The right reason to get yourself 'birded-up'

Us men should only start a relationship and get ourselves a girlfriend when we believe the girl in question could be the one we end up spending the rest of our life with. I know this sounds a bit heavy, but if we get into a relationship for the wrong reasons then it's unlikely the relationship will last, and all we'll end up with is headaches and a lot of wasted time and energy. Keep in mind, there's nothing wrong with staying single. Some of the happiest blokes I know are single. Next-door neighbour Dave is single, and when I asked him why he never got married he replied:

"Why eat steak 'n' 3 veg 7 days a week when you can feast from a smorgasbord every night?"

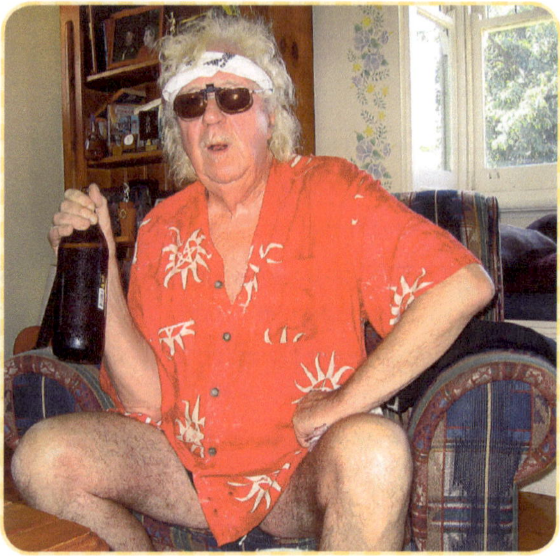

Chapter 20
Winning her over

Women may choose a husband for his money, they may choose him for his looks, but they can never really fall in love with a man until they have been captivated by his soul.

(Source: Author's mum)

Let's say we've met ourselves a nice lady in the real world or on the Net. We've had a few dates and we really dig the lady in question. It's come to a point where we'd really like to make the relationship more permanent. The problem is, we're not quite sure how to go about it.

I'm sure most of us blokes have heard the conventional wisdom about winning over a woman—stuff like showering her with chocolates or flowers, taking her out for dinners at fancy restaurants, yaddah, yaddah, yaddah. Conventional wisdom means that every other bloke out there is trying the same angles. Forget all that stuff, it's boring and predictable—and what happens if our date meets some other dude who takes her to a fancier restaurant, buys her better quality chocolates, bigger flowers? We're stuffed.

> ***Key point:*** If all we show women is our external qualities, then we give them no choice but to judge us based on those qualities.

The way to win her over is to use what I call the 'aces-in-the-pack strategy'. The aces are designed to show her our inner beauty, our spirit. Why? Because women may choose men based on external qualities, such as appearance, for one-night stands or a bit of a fling, but most of them need to see more when considering a man for a long-term relationship; most of them need a connection of the souls.

So we don't waste our money on chocolates, flowers and fancy restaurants. If we use the aces-in-the-pack strategy, it won't matter if we look like a drunkard shot out of a cannon or smell like we've just slept in a cabbage patch full of horse fertiliser; we show her our inner beauty, captivate her with our beautiful soul and we win her over.

The Ace of Diamonds — The artistic soul

Nothing makes a woman go ga-ga quicker than a man with an artistic soul. So how do we make her think we have a bit of culture about us? How do we make her feel that beneath an average-looking exterior we have the creative fires and burning passions of an artistic soul? We write her a poem. And that doesn't mean simply copying a Shakespeare sonnet word-for-word—it means doing it ourselves. And don't worry, it's not that difficult to do; it doesn't even have to rhyme.

Tip for writing a poem: Make your poem subtle, but powerful and passionate. Make it clear in the poem that you really like the lady you intend to give the poem to.

Another tip: Why not include a famous artist in your poem? That way the recipient will not only be blown away by the fact that you can write poetry but also by your knowledge of art, and she will think you both talented *and* cultured.

Here's a poem I whipped up which has worked a treat for me on more than one occasion. If you can't be stuffed writing your own then feel free to use this one.

ODE TO VINCENT

Vincent Van Gogh was a nutter
He cut off his ear
But he didn't need his ears to see
He had eyes
And if he were alive
He'd want to paint you
Especially your magnificent thighs

But Vincent is dead
So forget about him, my dear
It's my turn to paint you
And I've got both my ears

I'll paint your pearly whites
I'll paint your pretty toes
I'll paint your magnificent heaving breasts

You won't even have to pose
Just give me something to take home
Maybe your pantyhose

Every time I see your face
I thank God that I was born
I hope you don't mind me saying so
But you give me the almighty horn

What I'm trying to say
Is that you're the one I really dig
You stir something in my loins
You make me impossibly big.

The Ace of Hearts — The tortured soul

Women can't help falling in love with a tortured soul. It's in their nature to want to make everything better, to take away the pain. Us men can use this to our advantage. How? We learn a few lines from a particularly sad, melancholic or morose song and we sing them to her (I like to use 'Send in the Clowns'). Every now and then we let loose a wail. When we stop singing, we turn away from her with a pained look on our face. Guaranteed, she'll want to take us into a comforting cuddle and whisper a few soothing words in our ear.

The Ace of Clubs — The adventurous soul

Another potent method for winning a potential girlfriend over is to give her the sense that life with us would be an adventure. Does that mean dragging her off to do a little white water rafting or go–kart racing? No. Us blokes love adrenalin-charged activities, but most women's sense of adventure is not adrenalin based.

The key for us men in passing ourselves off as the adventurous type is symbolism. Women read lots of romantic fiction, and romantic fiction is full of adventurous male stereotypes and archetypal heroes such as The Lonesome Cowboy, The Officer and the Gentleman, The Pirate King and The Lord of the Jungle. Do we need to become any of these archetypes to impress the womenfolk? No. We just use a symbol to associate ourselves with one of the archetypes—a patch over the eye, a cowboy hat or a loincloth will do the trick nicely.

> ***Tip for success:*** Next time your potential girlfriend asks you over for dinner, turn up with a nice bot of vino and nothing on save a loincloth. When she opens the door to greet you, you hit her with your best Tarzan 'call of the wild'. For added effect, see if you can get hold of a chimpanzee for the night. Or why not ask your potential squeeze to meet you down at the beach or local lake for a picnic. She arrives in her car, you arrive on horseback carrying a well-stocked picnic hamper. Take her for a gallop to a secluded cove where the three of you can watch the sunset together. She will love your adventurous spirit.

The Ace of Spades — The 'connected' soul

The womenfolk out there often talk about feeling 'connected' to the man they love. Establishing a connection with a woman occurs over time and will only happen if we are willing to open up and discuss deep and meaningful issues, such as dreams and aspirations, as well as listen and encourage her when she opens up to us. Communication is the key. However, most of us blokes fail at establishing a connection with a woman that we really dig because we:

- Talk about ourselves all night.
- Talk about topics of no interest to her, such as football, Formula 1 or must-see Internet sites like Upskirtnurses.com.
- Don't listen.
- Look disinterested whenever she has something to say.
- Have usually had too much to drink.

I have developed a strategy to help us blokes overcome our inability to connect—I call it the 'A.R.S.E. strategy'.

The A.R.S.E strategy

ASK her to tell you her dreams and aspirations.
REMAIN silent while she answers. If you find it hard to listen then put a mental picture in your mind and focus on that. Nod your head occasionally and maintain solid eye contact.
SOLICIT more information about her dreams and aspirations. Women usually stop talking at some point to gauge your interest. At that critical point, you need to jump in with, "Go on, I'm really interested, tell me more." Get her to talk as much as possible about herself, and use avoidance tactics like going to the toilet to get out of talking about yourself (just in case you say something stupid). The more she talks to you and the more she thinks you're actually listening, the more connected she will feel.
ENCOURAGE her to aim for her dreams. Be positive and inspiring.

Tip for success: When practicing the A.R.S.E strategy, make sure you employ the correct listening skills—it is vitally important to always look interested when listening.

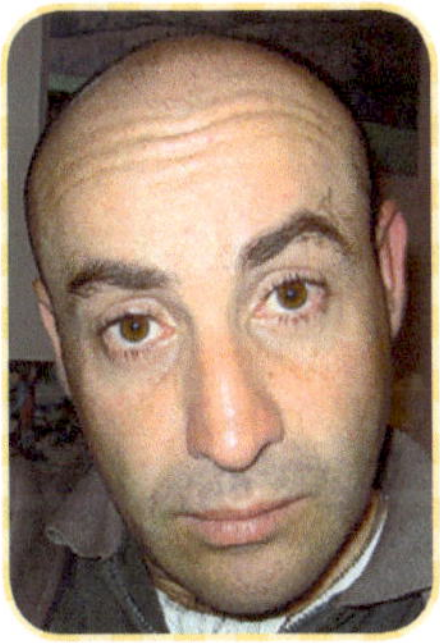

Yes!

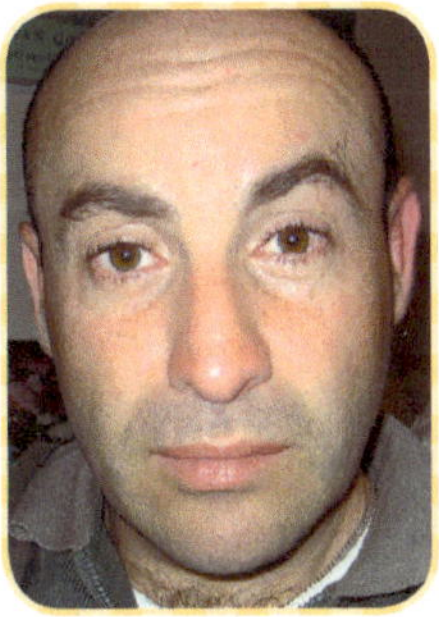

Yes!

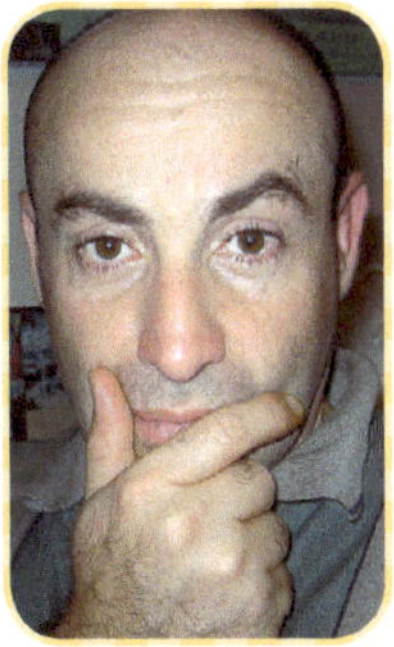

Yes!

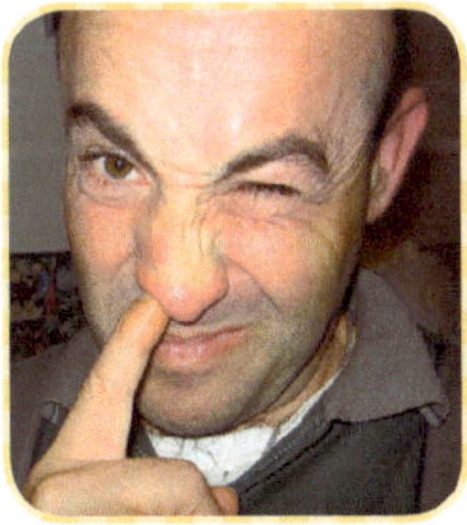

No!

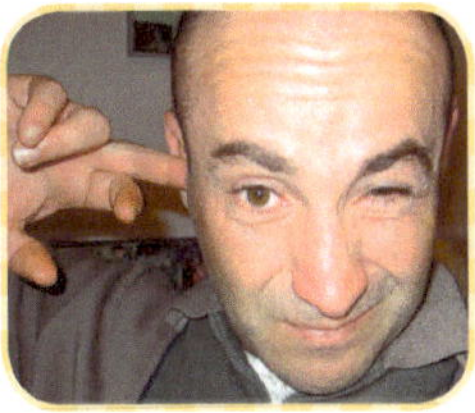

No!

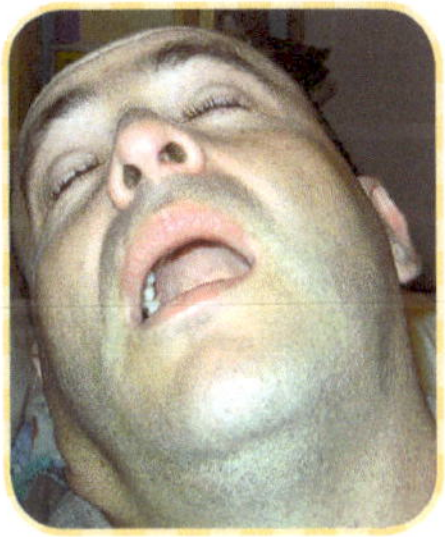

Definitely not!

In summary

Yes, people do get into relationships for money; they do get into relationships because they want to be with someone powerful or famous or handsome. But these relationships are unlikely to last, because external, superficial connections are unlikely to make a couple stick together through the hard times. It takes an internal connection of spirit to enable a couple to stand the test of time. Women understand this better than us men, and when they look for a potential partner, most of them look for the beauty inside. By using the aces, we can show the woman of our dreams our inner beauty and, in the process, form a powerful connection with her. Put simply, we use the aces to win her heart and her soul, and possibly get ourselves into a relationship that lasts.

Part 4 — Summary and conclusions

When we're teenage lads, relationships come and go like the latest fads, and we change our girlfriends as often as we change our underpants—at least once a week. But as we get older, getting in and out of relationships is a waste of time and money, and can result in a lot of unnecessary stress. We must be sure, when starting a relationship, that we're thinking of the lady in question as a potential life-partner and not a stop-gap until something better comes along. And if we are sure, we now have the knowledge to win her over. We can do it; we hold all the aces.

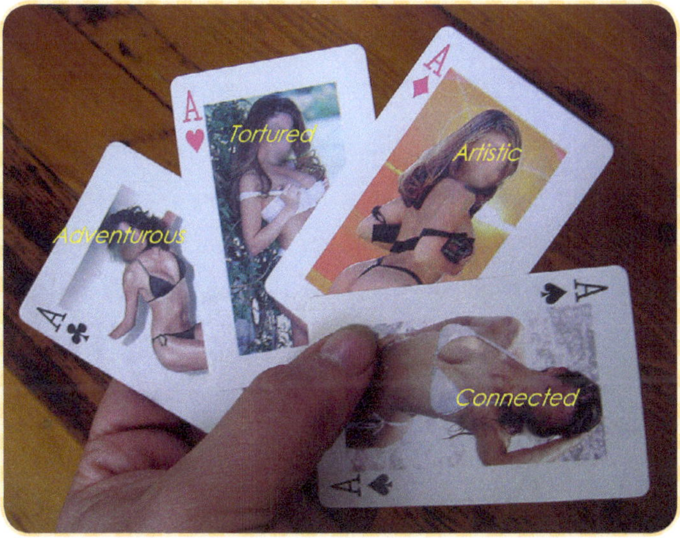
Adventurous
Tortured
Artistic
Connected

PART V

Fat and happy: The science of successful long-term relationships

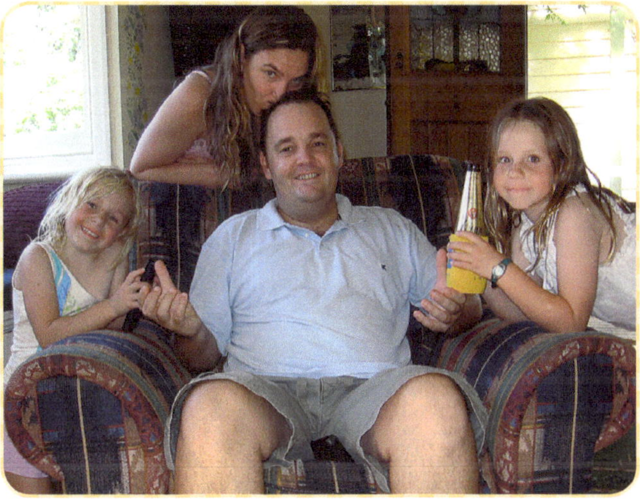

Chapter 21
Warning: There's a huge difference between a girlfriend and a wife

If there's a big difference between a casual relationship and a girlfriend, then there's an absolute Grand Canyon of a difference between a girlfriend and a long-term partner. So many relationships that bubble along happily as boyfriend/girlfriend fail miserably as fiancé/fiancé or partner/partner or husband/wife. Why? Because us blokes fail to seriously, and I mean seriously, consider the following questions: Am I really in love? Do I love her unconditionally? Am I ready to commit? Is she in love with me?

I'm not trying to scare anyone out of proposing (marriage is a wonderful state of being), but before us blokes get on bended knee, before we slip the ring on our lady-love's finger and crack open the bubbly, we must make sure we've got our heads around the following:

Am I in love?

How do us blokes know if we're in love? A lot has been written on this subject but most of the literature only serves to confuse. Allow me to simplify things with the following rule of thumb:

> ***A rule of thumb:*** Basically, if the end result of spending time with a woman is not simply a notch in the belt, then it may be love; but then again, it may just be friendship. If the lady we're spending time with leaves us experiencing a heady feeling of intoxication which makes us take leave of our senses, where she begins to occupy our thoughts to the point that other aspects of our life take second billing, then we may be experiencing 'crazy love', and we need to spend more time with the lady to discover whether we have 'unconditional love'.

Crazy love vs. Unconditional love

I'm sure we've all had a mate who's been rolling along happily single and then, bang, from out of nowhere he's hit fair and square between the shoulder blades by one of Cupid's crazy love arrows and he loses his friggin' marbles. He starts daydreaming, he spends less time with the boys, and when he does venture out he no longer wants to drink 10 pots of beer, puke and pass out, because he's going to the movies the next day with his lady-love to catch a double billing of *Breakfast at Tiffany's* and *Sleepless in Seattle*. And when he finally introduces the lady-love to the lads, the happy couple swoon over each other—calling each other pet names, hugging, kissing and talking like they're five-year-olds—to the point where it makes everyone else sick. Six months later they've broken up over some minor problem, like his habit of clipping toenails in the lounge room while watching sport.

Unfortunately, love is not all running hand-in-hand with our lady-love along a deserted beach, smiling wistfully at one another while humming Air Supply tunes. Love is hard work and requires effort. So the next time we spend a bit of time with a woman and start feeling a bout of the old 'crazy love' starting to take hold, we should pull our heads out of the clouds and ask ourselves the following questions:

a. If she doesn't get on with our best mates, who is more important to us?
b. If she drinks too much at a family do and ends up spewing all over the table in front of our parents, will we forgive her?
c. If she accidentally-on-purpose erases our porn collection with episodes of *Desperate Housewives*, will we get over it?
d. If she isn't interested in kids, cooking or keeping house, is that an issue?

The point I'm making here is that there are two kinds of love: 'crazy love' and 'unconditional love'. Unconditional love is where us blokes are prepared to love our partners no matter what. And that can only come with time, as we get to know them. So my advice for us blokes is to live with the woman that's captured our hearts for at least a year before we go making long-term plans.

Commitment — The 'C' bomb

Another idea that us blokes have trouble understanding—or choose to ignore—is the 'C' bomb. Why 'C' bomb? Because it is the one thing that continually blows up in our faces. Men just don't understand the concept of commitment. And that's probably a good thing, because if we did then none of us would get married in the first place.

Commitment means the following to a woman: sharing life completely with another human being, with both partners helping each other to be the best that they can be. Sounds harmless enough, don't it? But let me break it down into man-speak—we can no longer do what we want, whenever we want, to whomever we want.

The commitment test — Have you thought about the following?

- Am I ready to share the responsibility of looking after kids, as well as housework and other domestic duties, to ensure my partner has free time to pursue social activities and personal interests, just like I expect to be able to?
- Am I ready to support her in her academic or career pursuits just as I expect her to support me?
- Am I ready to call what's mine "ours" and set up joint financial and investment strategies?

No? You haven't thought about the above? I bet she has.

Gents, in this day and age, if we think we simply tie the knot, bring home the bacon and spend every Friday night getting pissed with our mates while the good lady wife does the shopping and vacuums the floor, then we had better think again. If we're still thinking in terms of 'I', and not 'we', then we're not ready to commit. Full stop!

Is she in love with you?

Believe it or not, women can be just as predatory as men. Sometimes we're so blinded by love (or lust) that we fail to pick up the signs that we're being strung along. We end up spending a whole lot of time and effort (and money) trying to win her heart, only to get dumped without explanation. An old Greek proverb sums it up nicely:

One pubic hair from a woman has the strength to tow a ship.

So how do us blokes know if our partners are really in love with us? How do we know if she's a keeper? There is only one sure-fire way to find out—I call it the 'toilet test'. The blokes in our family have been using this simple test for generations, and we haven't had one divorce yet.

The Toilet Test

If your woman is prepared to enter the toilet without complaining after you've stunk it up real good, marry the girl, because it's true love.

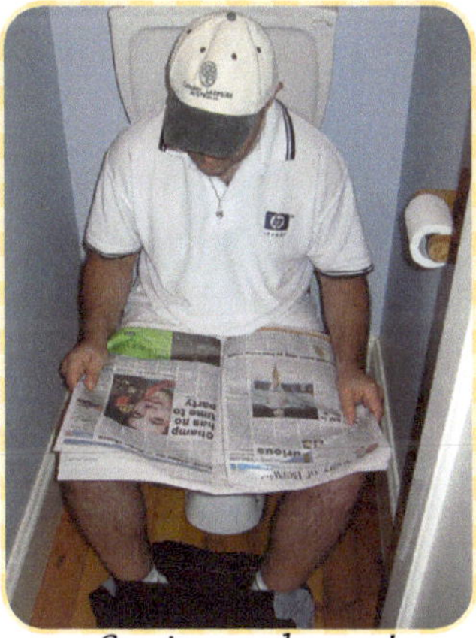

Setting up the test!

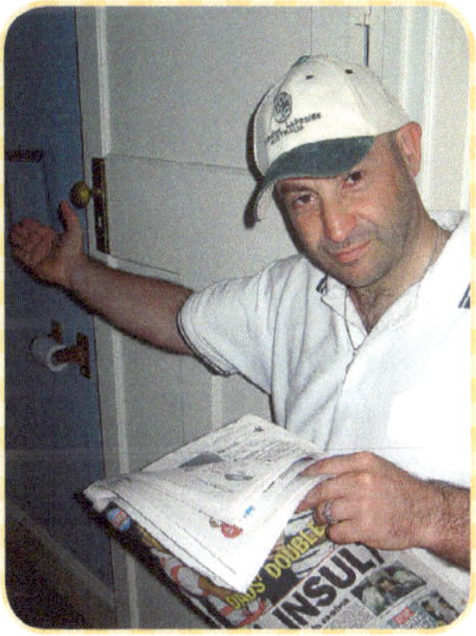

After you, love!

Chapter 22
Why do so many long-term relationships fail?

Despite what us men would like to believe, as soon as we get into a long-term relationship such as marriage, it's a whole new ball game. Trust me, things change. She changes, you change, your environment changes. And here's how:

She changes

Allow me to illustrate how she changes using the following scenario:

The 'just married' scenario

You've just announced to the world your intention to be life-partners, or jumped on the plane to Fiji after getting legless at your own wedding. What follows is a honeymoon period; a period during which everything is rosy, when you and your missus go at it day and night like a couple of baboons on heat, when nothing's a problem and everything's an adventure.

Then one day the honeymoon is over. It's like an invisible switch has been flicked on the missus and all of a sudden she starts talking like some alien. She starts using words and phrases like "priorities", "planning for the future", "upgrading the décor". She begins giving you directions—and just in case you don't understand the verbals, she writes them down for you (shopping lists, odd jobs lists, etc.). Out of nowhere she wants 20 multi-coloured pillows for the bed and a new couch, even though the old one does the job perfectly. Christmas cards and thank-you notes have now become a major priority. And heading over to a friend's house for a simple BBQ is no longer that simple: it is now a logistical nightmare of organising dips, nibbles, drinks, and "Who's bringing what?" and "Is this dress okay or should I wear the red one?"

She will try to change you

Women are much better at dealing with change than us men. In fact, for the most part, they love making changes, and we can be sure when they've done changing themselves and their environment they're going to have a crack at changing us.

Without warning, we'll notice that our favourite collection of 20-year-old undies and t-shirts have gone missing—replaced by designer Polos and funky hipster briefs. New business shirts appear in our wardrobe. Scented candles have replaced the stash of *Playboy* mags in the toilet. No matter how many times we tell her that we're happy going to our mate's BBQ in a singlet and shorts, she simply nods and smiles and says, "Of course, sweetie, but how about you wear the new shirt I bought you, and remember to keep your mouth closed and your elbows off the table when you eat."

Women aren't stupid, though; they won't try and change everything at once. No way. They'll do it slowly, subtly. They will try and change the way we behave, the way we look, and our priorities. The 'sisterhood' even has a phrase for this behaviour modification process—'breaking in your man'.

There are many reasons why our better halves will try to change us, and most of the time it's not because they're unhappy with us—they just want us to be better. They want to be proud of us. They want to be able to show us off in front of their girlfriends and gloat about how much they've improved us. They want to be able to say to the mother-in-law, "Look at what I've done with your boy, and you thought I wasn't good enough for him."

A woman's weapons for changing a man

1. Sex

Behaviour modification techniques using treats have been used to train animals since Moses was a boy—do what you're told and you get a treat, misbehave and you're denied the treat. Us men are no different to any other animal, and women know this. They can get us up off the couch and mowing the back lawn in a flash just with the promise of an afternoon knee-trembler on completion of the task.

2. The Social Diary

Make no mistake, the social diary is one of the most effective behaviour modification weapons that women have in their arsenal. It's an unwritten contract that's so effective because it works by stealth. Some women may use a plain old diary, while others will use a calendar. Either way, they will plan our whole year out for us in advance just by adding an entry next to a date.

A typical calendar negotiation discussion:

Us blokes:	"Oh, by the way, honey, Robbo and I are going to the game next weekend."
Our partners:	"Did you put it in the calendar?"
Us blokes:	"No. What calendar?"
Our partners:	"The one on the dishwasher. Just a sec, I'll check it and see if we're free."
Us blokes:	"I didn't realise —"
Our partners:	"Sorry, love, but we're going over to Mum's for dinner."
Us blokes:	"Your mum's? But ... hang on ... when did we —"
Our partners:	"It's in the calendar, sweetie, you can check it for yourself if you like."

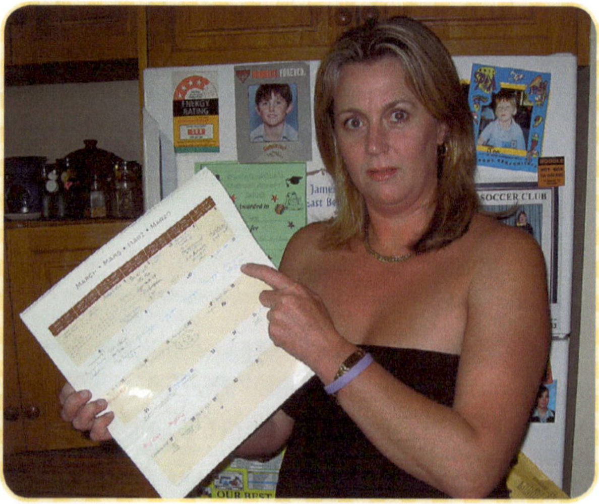

You change

These days, most of us men don't enter into long-term relationships expecting to remain the same person we were in our single days; we understand the need to give up some of our personal freedoms and luxuries. Some of us adapt to the changes, while others are not prepared for the volume of change and, as a consequence, react in two ways:

1. Become a dictator

In the face of such change, some men feel the need to stamp their authority on the relationship—"I wear the pants" type stuff. Rather than discuss and listen, they demand and order. Fifty years ago women put up with this type of behaviour, but not nowadays. I can just hear all those he-men out there saying, "Crap, I can do what I like. I've got my missus under control. It's all about keeping her under a tight reign." REALITY CHECK! While you're down at the pub with your mates, your missus is probably opening the door to the local pizza boy, purring like a kitten and dressed in her best lingerie.

2. Become a doormat

Overwhelmed by the volume of change, some men simply accept it and end up 'wearing the skirt' in the relationship. Men in this position often display behavioural patterns such as:

- Apologising even when they don't understand what they're apologising for.
- Feeling guilty about stuff they've previously never given a second thought about (like an afternoon nap in front of the telly).

- Feeling the need to justify their actions, when in days gone by they couldn't give a hoot what anyone else thought.
- Making excuses like "Just stepping out to get the milk, dear", just so they can get some time to go down to the local for a beer.

Women do not want doormats for partners; they don't want someone they can walk all over. Men who simply bow to all of their partner's demands will eventually lose her respect. Neither do women want dictators—men who are stubborn, threatening and loud, who insist it's their way or the highway.

In summary

As far as us men are concerned, most of our long-term relationships fail because we cannot deal with the volume of change taking place around us. As a consequence of this change, we feel as though we need to change ourselves to cope. And as a consequence of that, we end up feeling resentful for losing our identity. Once a man feels as though he has lost his identity in the relationship, it's all over, red rover.

Chapter 23
Why do relationships succeed?

I come across a lot of men experiencing relationship problems, and an increasing number of them are turning to daytime chat shows to get the good oil on how to put things right. Watching a few episodes of *Dr Phil* and taking on a bit of chat show wisdom don't mean our relationships will take a turn for the better. Why? Because these shows are predominately watched by women, and therefore display a strong bias towards the female point of view on relationships, so a lot of what's said just doesn't make sense or work for us blokes.

What us blokes need is advice straight from the horse's mouth; advice from experienced men who have been there, done that: men in happy long-term relationships who can give us guidance we can easily understand and put into practice. With this in mind, I recently had a chat to a group of Brits (pictured below) who visited the pub on the way to supporting their beloved British Lions take on the Aussies in rugby. Given that these blokes are away from home for extended periods of time, watching sport and drinking beer, and are still happily married, I decided to pick their brains and discover the key ingredients to successful long-term relationships.

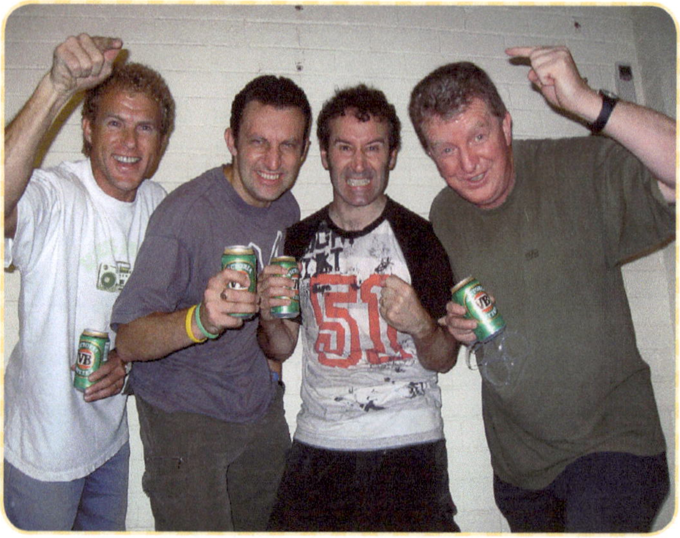

The lads giving me the good oil on what makes relationships last.

All the men I spoke to agreed that love is the foundation, the rock upon which a successful relationship is built. All of them agreed there must also be trust. But none of them mentioned the so-called 'big ticket' relationship items, such as negotiation, compromise, communication, quality time together, intimacy, openness and oneness. According to the blokes I spoke to, the key ingredients to successful long-term relationships are as follows:

- Reminding her every now and again that you wear the pants.

- Learning how to avoid conflict.
- Learning how to get that magical 'leave pass' the easy way.
- Learning how to get out of the dog house when you've stuffed up.
- Learning how to make sure that she only has eyes for you.

Chapter 24
Wearing the pants

Gents, there will be times in our long-term relationships when we'll need to stand up for ourselves and wear the pants. It won't happen that often—for the most part, most of us are happy to go along with whatever the missus decides or plans—but when it does happen, the only way we'll successfully make a stand without having to go through a heated argument or protracted negotiation is if we have the respect of our partners.

How do we get their respect? We don't get it through threats or violence. Neither do we get it by sitting on our fat arses all day while they do all the work. At the very least, we need to pull our weight around the place and contribute to the upkeep of the household. But if we *are* contributing and *still* find ourselves becoming a dictator just to get our own way, or giving in and becoming a doormat, then the following simple techniques may be helpful:

The raw steak technique

Don't believe all that crap about women preferring SNAGS (Sensitive New Age Guys). Sooner or later women get sick of all that sensitivity and want to be reminded they're going out with a 'real man'. They want to know that their man has the balls to stand up and protect them, should the need arise. Women will respect us if they feel we can protect them. And even if we don't have the balls, we can still make them think we do by showing them a glimpse of the 'savage within'.

How do we give them a glimpse of the savage within? We use the 'raw steak technique'. The next time your better half cooks you a steak, you ask for it raw and bloody. Forget the knife and fork, just pick it up off of the plate and start ripping into it; gnaw at it, chew, tear, make some dog noises and smear some blood over your face as you wipe your mouth. Trust me, she'll be impressed and unlikely to argue the point the next time you need to make a decision.

The stubborn mule technique

Every now and again, we men should take a relatively simple task and make it unnecessarily difficult. This could apply to any household task, but the easiest one to use is the 'unnecessary detour'. The next time we need to pack the family into the people-mover and go visit the parents-in-law, we use a few delaying tactics to make sure we're running late, and then once we're on the road we take a route that our significant others are not familiar with. Our partners are sure to know the quickest route to their parents place and will no doubt be fuming at us for taking the scenic route, especially since we're running late. The more they fume, the more detours we take. Eventually they'll give up. When we do arrive at the in-laws, we simply smile and say, "Now wasn't that a beautiful drive?" The next time we set our minds to doing a task our way, our partners will be unlikely to waste time on trying to change our minds.

The personal touch technique

Most women have a nesting instinct (not all women, though). They like to take control of arranging the nest so that it's both fashionable and functional. For example, they will have firm ideas on how the house and garden should look, including colour schemes, furnishings and so on. It is important that us men add our own personal touches to whatever our partners arrange. If they create an English cottage garden theme in the front yard, then we go and grab ourselves a dirty great big Mexican cactus and plant it right smack bang in the middle of the garden. If they organise a Japanese garden theme in the backyard, then a well-placed golf practice net and a few ugly garden gnomes won't go astray. If they want the house decorated with abstract art, then we go purchase a big moose head and mount it where they can see it. No matter what our partners say, we act like we're really proud of our personal touches; and most importantly, we refuse to replace them at all costs. These items will be a constant reminder to our partner that we're no pushover.

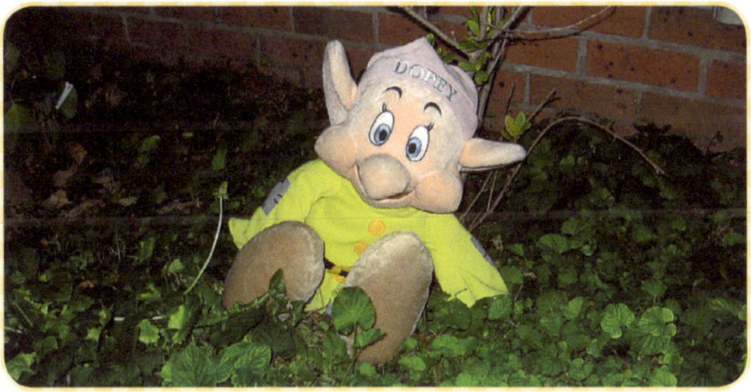

Chapter 25
Learning to avoid conflict

Every long-term relationship has its fair share of conflict. The way us men handle that conflict goes a long way to determining our happiness in the relationship. Modern relationship gurus advise us to approach any conflict with our partners in a rational way, reaching a resolution through plenty of open and honest dialogue. I disagree, however, and have found that most men in happy relationships don't tackle conflict head on, they avoid it.

Arguments are like seagulls: feed them and more will come. All you'll hear is a lot of loud squawking, all you'll be left with is shit everywhere. But if you ignore them they will eventually go away and shit somewhere else.

(Source: Unknown)

The art of listening without listening

The problem with arguments is that people, both men and women, are not used to conflict, and in the heat of the moment they often say things they don't mean and often regret. So how do we avoid arguing with our partners and potentially damaging our relationships? We practice the art of listening without listening.

Men who are happy in their relationships are adept at tuning in and out of conversations with their partner, which allows them to pick up what they need to know and ignore all the noise. How is this possible? Think of your daytime soap operas—you can miss a couple of days here and there and still be up to speed on the overall plot. Why? Because soap operas are repetitive and cover the same ground over and over again. It's the same deal with arguments.

The tune-in, tune-out technique

The next time we find ourselves in an argument with our partner, we take a deep breath and picture ourselves on a tropical island, sitting on a sun-chair while a bevy of bikini-clad beauties whistling the chorus to 'Don't Worry, Be Happy' bring us coconut shells filled with our favourite cocktail. We keep this image in mind for 20 seconds (careful not to lose ourselves and smile, or whistle along to the tune). At all times we maintain eye contact with our partner so she feels she has our absolute attention, even though we're millions of miles away. When the 20 seconds has elapsed, we allow ourselves to come back to reality for 20 seconds. We maintain this process of alternating between two worlds for 20 second periods until, after a while, our calm and composed demeanour will take the wind out of her sails. She'll eventually give up picking a fight and the argument will blow over. The next day, she won't even remember why she was angry with us in the first place. Happy days!

Small victories

Rather than trying to win every battle that comes our way in our relationships, us blokes should focus on the ones that we really want to win, and allow our partners to win the rest. Allowing her small victories will provide us with leverage when we need to push for something that is really important to us.

The small victories technique

If she wants to get a $300 haircut, then we let her. If she wants to be the decision maker—in regard to gifts for friends, holiday destinations, restaurants to eat at, movies to see—we let her. However, we only 'give in' after making a token display of resistance, occasionally throwing our arms up in the air and, with resignation, saying, "Okay, sweetheart, do what you want." When it comes time for us to push for something we really want, we gently remind her of all the times we've given in to her wishes. And then we can go out and purchase that ridiculously expensive piece of machinery that we've always wanted but will hardly ever use.

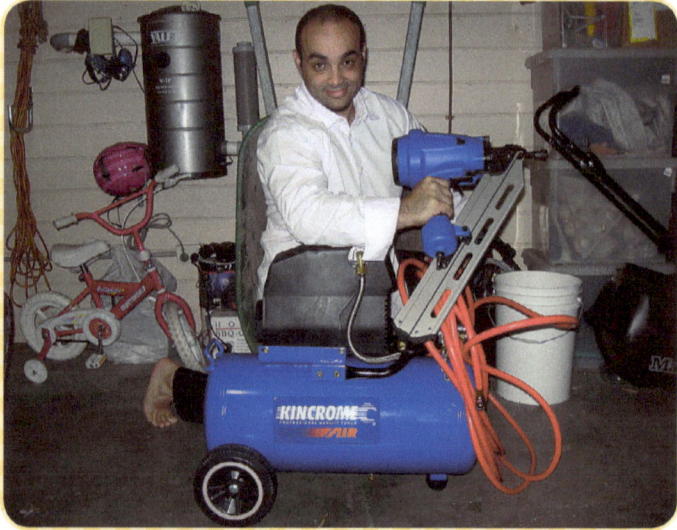

The author's brother looking super proud of himself after using the 'small victories technique' to negotiate his way to a brand new kick-arse compressor and nail gun combo — well done, tiger!

Chapter 26
The magical 'leave pass'

For those of us in long-term relationships, the 'leave pass' is truly a magical thing. Sure, there are plenty of blokes out there who don't feel the need to ask their partner's permission to go out with the lads, but that kind of attitude doesn't typically impress the missus and sooner or later it will cause problems in the relationship.

Wouldn't it be nice if we could turn to our partners and say, "I'm going away fishing this weekend and I'm going to drink lots of beer," only for them to reply with, "Sure, sweetie, catch a big one for me and have fun." Such an exchange is not beyond the realms of possibility. But make no bones about it, the unconditional approval of our partners for us men to go out and do what we want is not an easy ticket to purchase, yet it is an essential one for our happiness and well-being in long-term relationships.

LPI — The Leave Pass Index

Let's think of ourselves as having a Leave Pass Index. The LPI works in much the same way as any other index, indicating a positive or negative position. Most of us men would think the following would ensure a positive LPI:

- Sharing the domestic duties.
- Regular intimacy and communication.
- Remembering our partner's birthday and our anniversary.
- Bringing in a stable income.
- Buying her the occasional gift.
- Taking her out for the occasional dinner.

Performing the above would only give us a neutral LPI. Why? Because women expect us to do these kinds of things anyway, and they're unlikely to grant us a leave pass just because we do what is expected. If we want to boost our LPI, we need to extend our repertoire a little and do the unexpected.

Boosting our LPI

Wash her hair

Women love their hair being washed by a pair of hands other than their own; the experience is both intimate and sensual. Every now and again us blokes should offer to do the honour; it doesn't take much effort on our part and our LPI will skyrocket as a result. But we must be careful not to undo all our good work by pointing out imperfections, like grey hairs, split ends or dandruff. And we shouldn't go about it as though we're fossicking for gold—long, slow and smooth strokes are the only way to do it.

Write her an intimate letter

As women get older they become more and more insecure about their attractiveness. So, every once in a while (or whenever we're in desperate need of a leave pass), us fellas should take the time to remind our partner she is still the object of our desire by writing her an intimate letter. We should make it quite clear in the letter that we find her even sexier now than when we first met.

> ***Tip for success:*** Spice your letter up a bit by using erotic and sensual language—if you haven't got a clue about how to write in erotic and sensual language, then check out the Forum section in *Penthouse*. If you still haven't got a clue, then below is a sample letter I've knocked up. Feel free to use it.
>
> *Dearest Rosemary,*
>
> *After 10 years together, you still take my breath away. Even now when you bend over to pull out the weeds, dressed in your old trakky-daks, I get an aching in my loins that no amount of aspirin could get rid of. Though you've had two kids, you still have an hour-glass figure—even if the sands of time have become jammed in the wrong places. When I watch you doing your aerobics, dressed in your favourite bike pants, I am hypnotised by your buttocks, the two hemispheres gently nudging one another as you jog on the spot, like two baby elephants gently play-fighting in a tent.*
>
> *And oh how I love to watch you sleep. You look so beautiful, still comatose after a big night on the turps. The sound of your snoring is like the mating call of a moose, and the powerful melody is enough to start a stirring in my pyjama pants. And when finally you do rise and head for the shower, I often follow and just watch you soaping up, rejoicing in your natural glory, your red hair wet and slick, your breasts*

glistening like a couple of soccer balls kicked over wet grass, and your expertly manicured patch of rust-coloured down nestled between your milky thighs ... Yes ... Yes ... You are my fire-crotch, and the sight of you naked is enough to make my manhood begin to dance, rising and swaying like a cobra to the sounds of a flute. Yours is the only tune my cobra will ever dance to, my darling—yours, and yours alone.

Allow her to take time out

Another powerful strategy to boost our LPI is to give our partner the opportunity to take some time out. Time out is like gold to the womenfolk, especially if there are rugrats to look after. Us blokes should encourage our partners to spend some time by themselves recharging the batteries. There are lots of ways to do this—give her a full day of pampering at the local health spa, for example. But if we really want the best bang for our buck in terms of LPI then we organise a weekend away for the missus and her girlfriends, making sure we also ship off the kids for a visit to the grandparents. She gets time out, we get the house to ourselves; and the next time we want a weekend away with our mates, we get the green light with no complaints.

Cook her dinner

We should never underestimate the positive effects of cooking our partner a meal every once in a while. To most women, the sight of a man in the kitchen is like spotting a UFO—unexpected, mind-boggling, hard-to-believe and out of this world. A man who cooks impresses the hell out of them, and we don't need to be 5-star chefs to whip up something special. In any case, it doesn't really matter what gastronomic delights we prepare—it doesn't even matter if we stuff up and burn the hell out of whatever we're cooking—our partner will still think we're special because we've made the effort.

Handy hint: You can really tart-up an ordinary meal by announcing it in French and throwing in some garnishes.

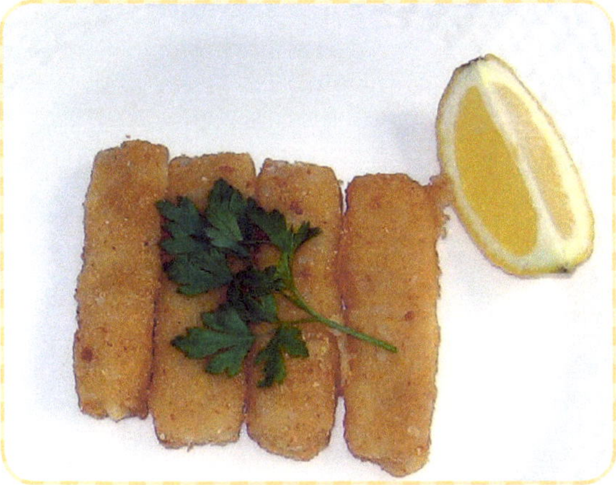

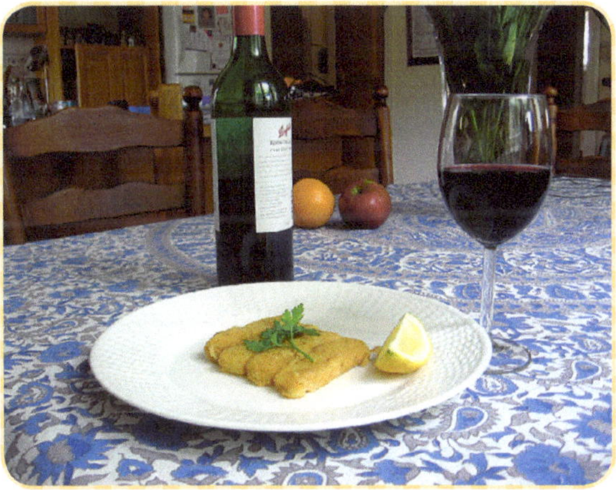

The author's signature dish — Doigts des poisons garnished with fresh parsley and a wedge of lemon — Bon Appetit!

Buy her a gift

Us men have no clue when it comes to the importance of gift giving. We can have done all the right things, only to watch helplessly as our LPI plummets because of a lazy last-minute attempt at a present. On the other hand, we can have underperformed all week and still send our LPI soaring with a well thought out gift. Here are some general rules of thumb for gift giving:

a. Don't kid yourself, women want jewellery

That's right, we blokes hear lots of rubbish about how "it's the thought that counts". Crap! Nothing gets a woman going like the glint of gold. At least once a year us blokes should go out and buy our beloved a decent piece of jewellery. It doesn't have to be ridiculously expensive, but we don't have to be cheap-skates, either. There is a wide variety to choose from these days, to suit every budget, from gold, diamonds and pearls, to birthstones, rings, pendants and chains. Even if we're struggling for a bit of coin we can still buy her something that's relatively cheap but looks fantastic. Remember—diamonds may be a girl's best friend, but cubic zirconias are a man's prayers answered.

b. Unexpected gifts

Most of us wait for a special occasion to buy our partner a gift: birthdays, anniversaries, Valentine's, Christmas and so on. Does this boost our LPI? No, because women expect gifts on these special days. What women don't expect is their menfolk to come home with an unexpected gift—one that's given for no other reason except to say "I love you". It doesn't even have to be an expensive gift: a book, movie tickets, a night out, flowers, chocolates, a plant, whatever. Women love it when we do this kind of stuff, and our LPI will go through the roof. (Warning: don't go overboard on the prezzies, otherwise you may set yourself a benchmark that's difficult to maintain.)

c. Think about it

I know a guy who bought his missus some anti-wrinkle cream for her birthday, and then followed it up with an expired lotto ticket for Valentine's. And he wonders why he finds it so hard to get a leave pass. Just as athletes have a banned substance list, so too us men should have a banned gift list. The items on this list should include:

- Anything that would make her feel like she's not perfect: a Wonderbra, for example, or a lose weight/get fit video.
- Anything that you think would make her (or your) life easier: a vacuum cleaner, a washing machine or a dust-buster.
- Anything that can be used by the whole family: a computer, an Ipod, a TV.
- Novelty items such as alarm clocks that scream "WAKE UP, HONEY, IT'S TIME FOR BREAKFAST!", or the battery-operated-toy-man-in-a-trench-coat who exposes himself and shouts "Happy Birthday, Baby!"
- A wad of cash with a note that says 'Go choose your own present'.
- Jewellery that's made with beads, leather straps or alloy metals.

d. If in doubt, ask her

We all like to surprise our partners, but how often does the surprise really pay off? More often than not, our significant other receives our gift, tries hard to look pleased and then, as soon as our back is turned, rushes down to the hallway closet to stash it with all the other useless gifts we've bought her. Asking our partners what they want means that our presents will always hit their mark. However, we must make sure we get as many details as possible. This is especially true when buying clothes—we wouldn't want to buy her something that would look better on her mother (or grandmother, God forbid!).

e. Gifts that work are the ones that stir feelings

If Valentine's Day is around the corner or an anniversary is approaching and we want to pull out all the stops to get our missus something special, then we choose a gift that's personal in nature; one that she'll understand is just for her and not everyone else in the family; one that will stir her emotions. Personal gifts that work include items such as jewellery set with her birthstone, a painting of her favourite place, or a video/CD of your life together. Personal items that don't work include t-shirts emblazoned with slogans such as 'World's Best Wife' or 'I can't cook, I can't clean, but my man is happy coz I'm a sex machine'.

In summary

An unconditional leave pass is a vital ingredient in a happy long-term relationship for us blokes. If we simply do what's expected of us then our chances of scoring one are slim to none; but if we embrace just a few of the simple strategies mentioned above, then getting a night out with the lads becomes a relatively stress-free exercise. If we embrace all of the strategies, the next time we want to go away on a weekend of drunken debauchery with our mates, not only will our significant other send us away with a smile and a kiss, she'll probably pack our Esky for us as well. How good is that?

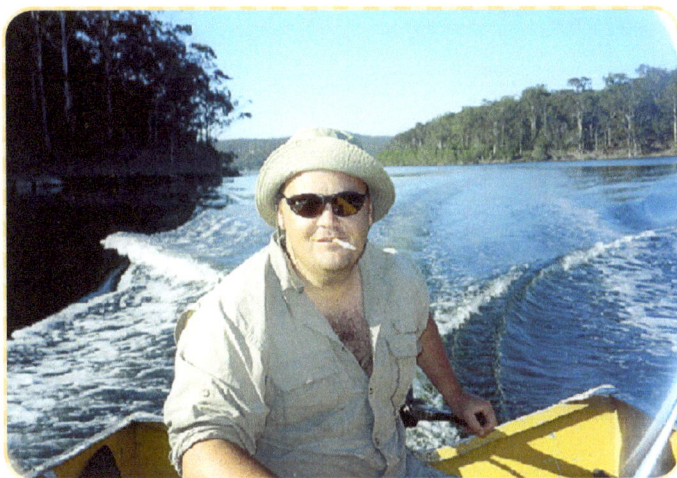

Get yourself that magical 'leave pass' and this could be you.

Chapter 27
Getting out of the dog house

Sooner or later, in any long-term relationship, us men find ourselves stuffing up. Stuff-ups can occur on a minor scale—leaving dirty clothes and dishes all over the place, farting in bed, or forgetting to bring home the milk and bread. Or they can be major ones—arriving home drunk at some ungodly hour, flirting with our partner's best friend, forgetting our partner's birthday or our wedding anniversary. Our minor stuff-ups are usually forgotten very quickly, but the major ones almost always result in a trip to the dog house.

Men who are happy in their relationships accept the fact that they will end up in the dog house every now and again. They don't worry about it too much because they know the secret to getting out. And what is the secret? Flowers and an apology won't do it; neither will chocolates. There's really only one way to go about it and it's deceptively simple; best of all, it doesn't involve any form of begging or grovelling. All we need to do to get ourselves out of the dog house is give our partner a foot-massage.

Don't believe me? Listen up—WOMEN DREAM OF GETTING THEIR FEET MASSAGED. Why? Two reasons. Firstly, because the feet are a Disneyland of nerve-endings and receptors, and a lot of women spend most of the day on their feet, often wearing high heels. Imagine how their feet must feel at the end of the day, and imagine the sheer bliss they would experience from a simple foot rub.

The second reason is that the massaging of the feet is one of the most intimate acts a woman can experience. Most of us blokes turn our noses up at the thought of massaging our partner's feet, but that's only because we don't understand the benefits, which are twofold. One, because foot massages are so intimate, those of us who aren't touchy-feely types can give our partners their intimacy fix all in one go, avoiding the need for all that hand-holding and cuddling bizzo, leaving our hands free for all the important stuff, like operating the remote. Two, the feet are an erogenous zone, and giving our partners a foot massage is likely to turn them to jelly; as a result, they'll forgive any indiscretions we may have committed with a few "ooohs" and "aaahs", polished off with an "I forgive you, baby, just keep massaging my feet."

Tip for success: If your missus has got manky feet, then use surgical gloves for the procedure and place cotton wool in your nostrils — it's a small price to pay for freedom from the dog house.

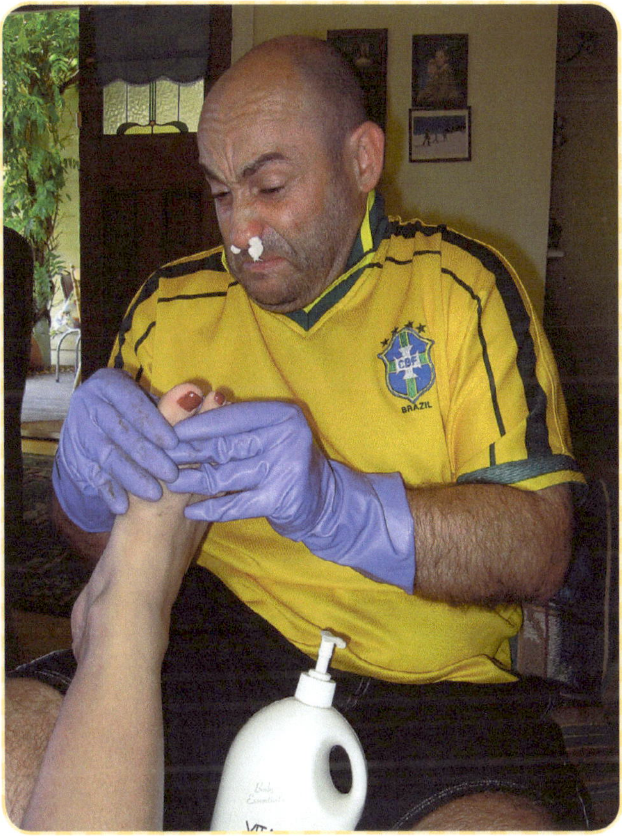
BRAZIL

Chapter 28
Making sure she only has eyes for you

Men in happy relationships are not only secure in their identity but also in the knowledge that their partners only have eyes for them. These men are able to go out with their partner and not feel the need to sneak a few peaks over the shoulder just to make sure everything is in order. And they have no problems letting their partner go on a girl's night out. In other words, these men are not slaves to the 'green dragon' of jealousy; and that is the ideal situation, because insecurity over our partners will ultimately lead to problems, and problems will not make us men happy.

So how do we make sure our lady-love is not closing her eyes and thinking of Johnny Depp the next time there's a bit of work being done between the sheets? The answer—be spontaneous, be sexy, and stuff up occasionally.

Spontaneity

Relationships fall into a pattern as they mature. The pattern is usually based around logistics, such as kids' soccer practice, shopping nights, school plays, and so on and so forth. The problem is that people get bored with routine, and after a while the constant drag of doing the same ol' same ol' can make one or both partners start to wonder whether the grass is greener on the other side of the fence. If us blokes want to make sure our partners are not the ones looking over the fence then we need to take the lead in putting some spice back into our relationships. Here are some simple ways to do it:

a. The slap on the ass

I'm not advocating we step up and whack her rump like we're trying to hit a ball out of the park. Don't cup and don't pat, either. The best method is to give our partner one swift and firm slap on the ass when she's not expecting it, and then walk away smiling mischievously.

b. The couple that washes together, stays together

Showering these days has become a mechanical process instead of a pleasurable experience. Next time our partner jumps in the shower, we jump in there with her and give her a real good lathering. We should be theatrical about it—beat our chest, roar, sing. She'll love us for it.

Tip for success: Even better than showering together is bathing together. Next time your missus goes to jump in the shower, you gently hold her back and tell her you've got a better idea (she'll think you're crazy, but push on). Begin filling the bath tub and then throw in a few of the rose petals that you nicked from the neighbour's garden. Add some scented oils and then assist her to get into the tub. Then jump in yourself (resist the urge to fart, fondle the crown jewels or clean your butt while you're in there). She'll think you're great.

c. Get her out of the house

The last thing us blokes want to do on a weekend while we're kicking back enjoying *World's Funniest Sports Bloopers — Volume 19* on channel 351 is leave our comfy armchair to head down to a windswept beach for a romantic stroll. But unlike us, women need to get out of the house. So we check the weather channel and we wait until we get a weekend with a strong possibility of rain. Just before the deluge is due to hit, we make a show of throwing down the remote and then turn to our beloved and say, "Sweetheart, grab some wine and a blanket and let's go down to the beach for a snuggle." She'll love our spontaneity, and we'll be back in that comfy armchair in the blink of an eye.

Tip for success: Just in case the weather channel gets it wrong, leave a door, tap or an electrical appliance on, or a window open, before you leave the house; that way you always have an excuse to come home early and catch *World's Funniest Sports Bloopers — Vol 20*.

Sex appeal

Us men think it's our God-given right to get fat and lazy as soon as the ink is dry on the wedding certificate. Hell, we've done all the hard work to get our girl and now it's time to kick back, relax and enjoy the green grass of the retirement paddock. Problem is, sooner or later we wake up and realise we can't see our toes as we shower on account of the bulging roof over the toolshed, and our missus no longer looks at us with that certain twinkle in her eye. We start to worry and decide we need to get ourselves back into shape, only to realise after the first 10 metres of a jog that the body is not what it used to be.

Quite mistakenly, most of us blokes think improving our physical appearance is the only way to get back lost sex appeal. Wrong. Sex appeal is not just about physical attributes, it's also about attitude. What's the right attitude? It's thinking 'sexy' whenever we do anything. Allow me to illustrate.

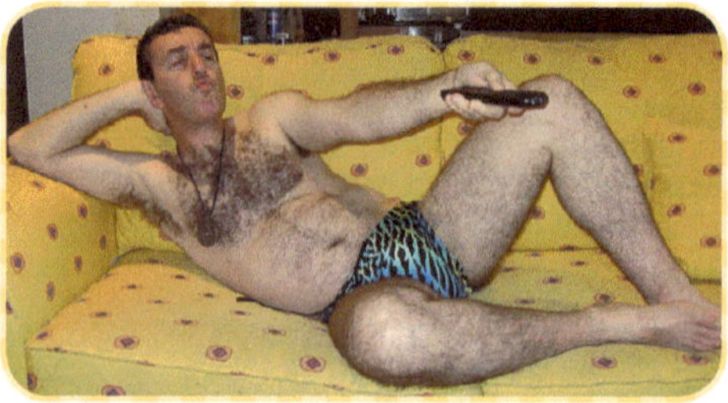

Watching TV and looking sexy.

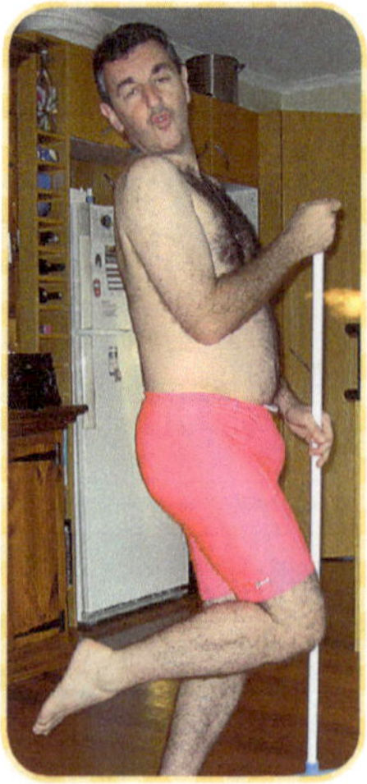

Sweeping, and still sexy.

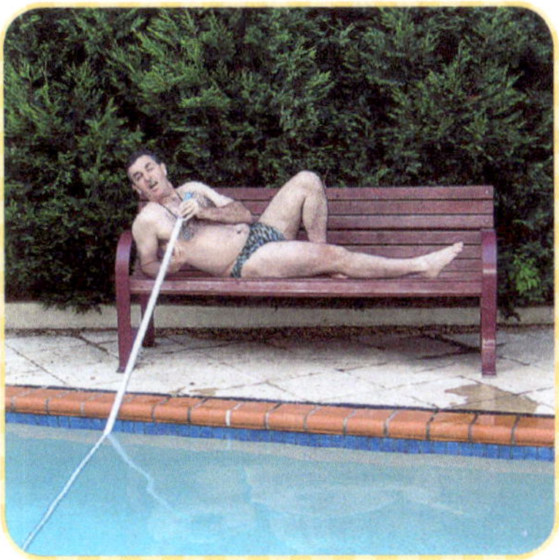

Cleaning the pool sexy.

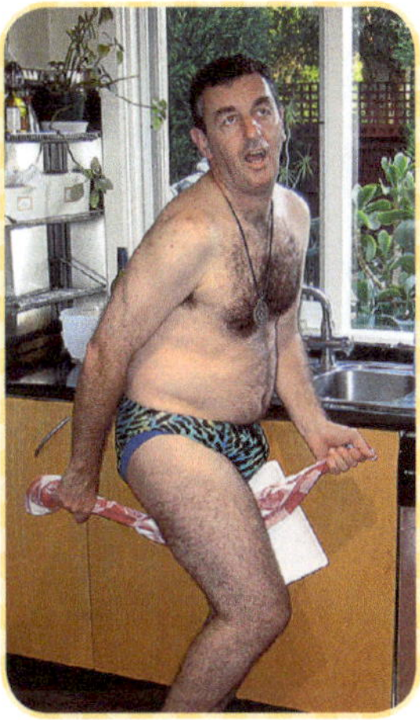

Drying the dishes — dead sexy!

Stuff up occasionally

Women are unlikely to stray from men who make them laugh. A good sense of humour is one of the most attractive qualities us men can possess. The problem is, very few of us are blessed with comedic talent; but if we can't be funny, why not be endearing? It's the next best thing. Hugh Grant is a classic example: the ladies love him because he's not perfect. He stuffs up, and his stuff-ups are endearing. How do we become endearing? We stuff up occasionally just like Hugh.

How to stuff up endearingly

- We have a go at washing the clothes. We make sure there's nothing in the wash that she loves (or we love) and then we mix the colours in with the whites.

- We invite the in-laws over for the Sunday roast, telling everyone that we'll be doing the cooking, and then we burn the crap out of it!
- We buy something that's DIY assembly and then assemble it all wrong. When we're finished, we call everyone over and unveil it theatrically and with a great sense of pride, making sure that it doesn't look anything like it's supposed to or it breaks soon after assembly.

Tip for success: To get the most sympathy mileage, wait until everyone laughs at your stuff up and then manufacture a mildly dejected, suitably embarrassed look. Guaranteed, your partner will give you a warm, comforting hug and say, "It's okay, sweetie, at least you tried."

Chapter 29
Sex for men in long-term relationships

The first few years of a long-term relationship are the halcyon years in the sex lives of us men. There's no longer any pressure to compete with other men; we can saddle-up and have sex any time of the day or night, as many times as we want (as long as our partner is up for it as well). All in all, life is good.

However, as our relationship matures, a strange quirk of nature kicks in and, even though we have the opportunity to have as much sex as we want, we no longer feel the need. Why?

Mother Nature's last laugh

The male sex drive is at its peak from our late teens to early twenties, whereas women don't hit overdrive until their early thirties. So us men spend the early part of our relationships on a sexual high, behaving like sex-crazed robots, tapping our partners on the shoulder day and night for a bit of nooky, saying stuff like, "You married a stud, baby, a sex machine." BUT as soon as we hit thirty-ish, everything changes, and then it's our better half in bed all dolled-up and ready for a bit of rumpy-pumpy, while the only pumping we're capable of is the snores out of our noses. We therefore leave our partner no option but to let out a frustrated, "Sex machine? Stud? Yeah, right," before rolling over, turning off the bedside lamp and dreaming of the young and virile photocopier technician back at work.

I like to call this strange quirk of nature 'Mother Nature's last laugh'.

Mother Nature's last laugh

Mother Nature gives us men the chemicals and hormones in our youth to make us think we are going to be indestructible sex gods for the rest of our lives, only to take them away from us and give them to our partners and wives so they can have the last laugh and forever remind us of our once much-vaunted sexual prowess. This is a clever scheme, on Mother Nature's behalf, to keep us blokes in check, for if The Horn ran riot in our bodies up until we died, none of us would ever settle down.

My libido ain't what it used to be

Along with a nose-diving sex drive, there are other factors in a maturing relationship that can impact the level of desire in us men—career concerns, kids and the mortgage, just to name a few. Plus, as we get older the stimuli that excite us sexually begin to change. Where once the sight of a bikini-clad beauty was enough to send us into meltdown, as we get older the sensory stimuli begin to have less effect but the mental stimuli become more powerful; that is, thoughts, memories and fantasies. That doesn't mean that a bikini-clad beauty won't excite us as we get older, but get her to open the fridge and bend down to pull out a few beers from the bottom shelf while dressed in a French maid's uniform, or pretend that she's our old high school teacher returned to punish us for being a bad boy, and guaranteed we'll be so worked up, steam will be coming out our ears.

Problem is, most blokes in long-term relationships aren't adventurous enough to ask their partners to indulge in a little role-play (or too embarrassed; because, let's face it, us blokes can dream up some really bizarre fantasies—one of my mates likes his partner to dress up as an Eskimo woman while he dons the polar bear gear. Go figure!). And in any case, most men in long-term relationships had their fun when they were young, and now they're ready for 'no-frills' sex once or twice a week. BEWARE! While us men approach our mid-life with a declining sex-drive, our partners and wives are approaching it like smouldering volcanoes of lust, ready to explode.

My missus knows more about sex than I do

Yep, us blokes don't get together with our mates and discuss sex. We may make a few lewd comments here and there, indulge in a bit of bragging, but in the main we talk about blokey stuff—cars, sport, work and so on. Meanwhile, our partners are out with the girls downing a few daiquiris and discussing the latest *Cosmo* 'sealed section' and celebrating the discovery of another erogenous zone. That's right, women discuss sex; and not only do they discuss sex, they love to get into the nitty-gritty. And there's plenty for them to discuss, because these days women's magazines seem to be discovering new erogenous zones with the same frequency that scientists discover new planets.

This can only result in our embarrassment when, after one of their daiquiri-drinking, sex-talking nights out with the girls, our partner returns home all hot and sweaty and ready for some luvin', and mid-coitus starts moaning demands and requests that include words such as G-spot and U-spot; telling us to bite here, put more pressure there; screaming at us to pull out the Osaki dolphin or the beads. All of which leaves us dazed and confused, wondering what the hell an Osaki dolphin is and which alien nation has abducted our wife.

> **Key point:** You may think you know all there is to know about sex; you may think you did all the necessary experimentation and exploration in your single days to make you a shag-meister—BUT YOUR'E WRONG. Your missus probably knows as much, if not more, than you do.

So how do us blokes in long-term relationships keep abreast of the ever-evolving sexual landscape? How do we satisfy the growing sexual appetites of our partners without sacrificing our comfort and routine?

If she's in the mood and you ain't

Unfortunately, more often than not, the last thing us men think about after a hard day's work is love-making. By the time we've had dinner, put the kids to bed, paid a few bills and completed various other odds and sods, we've got no energy left. Sure, our partners have probably completed a hard day's work as well, but thanks to Mother Nature's last laugh they're purring like kittens, ready for anything, while we're on the couch attempting to watch the TV through our eyelids. And should the good lady wife try to get our pistons pumping by donning the corset and crotchless panties, all we can do is respond with a tired, "Put that away, sweetie, I'm knackered." If that's the case then why not try the following:

1. **Get her to talk dirty to you**

Dirty talk is a massive turn on for us men, but most women find it a little embarrassing, or lack the knowledge and vocabulary to deliver the smut that gets our lust-O-meter redlining. However, with a little encouragement we can have our partners talking more filth than a sailor with Tourette's.

Tip for success: Next time you're in bed, throw the missus your favourite adult mag and ask her to read you a bedtime story. Better still, get her to add a few sound effects while she reads; maybe even play-out some of the actions. Sounds simple, doesn't it? Guaranteed, you'll be ready for action before she's even finished a page. And the beauty of this technique is that you can do it lying down with your eyes closed. Maximum return, minimum effort!

Why does this technique work so well? Because as us men get older, as our relationships become routine, fantasy plays a large part in what turns us on; what we imagine, not what we see, is the turn-on. Our missus reading us a paragraph about two nurses dressed in body-hugging latex uniforms sponge-bathing a man with a broken leg, coupled with her throwing in a few "oohs", "aahs" and "yeah baby's", along with a well-placed thermometer, will have us chomping at the bit like sex-starved stallions.

2. Spice things up a bit

Imagine if we turned up at work and picked up the phone to find that our first voicemail is a breathy message from the wife; something along the lines of:
"M-e-o-w, purr, m-e-o-w, purr ... Don't work late ... Kitty is waiting."

Encouraging the missus to leave suggestive voicemails, or e-mails, is one way to spice thing up. 'Dressing up' is another. Us blokes should get ourselves down to the local costume shop and grab some gear. Here are some very erotic costume combinations (the best combinations are those that require props).

- The aristocratic lord and the tavern wench.
- The kinky clown and the lion tamer's assistant.
- The naughty nun and the cheeky choir boy.
- The lusty cowboy and Pocahontas.

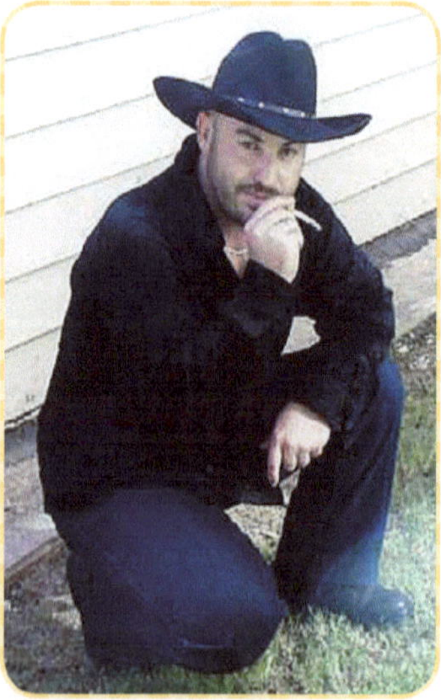

The author on a romantic week-end away with the missus, getting ready for a bit of cowboy v indian action. Giddyup!

Trust me, it's worth the effort. Remember, as we get older the brain becomes the most powerful sexual organ. Imagination is a far greater stimulant than physical reality. And don't think for one minute the wifey won't get into it; she'll love it, and so will you.

Handy hint: There are certain female characters that drive us blokes insane with lust—Wonder Woman, Barbarella, Ginger or Marianne (and maybe Mrs Howell for all the freaks out there). By far, one of the most popular is Genie of *I Dream of Genie* fame; and why not? What red-blooded male amongst us wouldn't be in seventh-heaven with a drop-dead gorgeous minx, who has magical powers, at our beck and call. So rather than buying your partner golf lessons or a bottle of perfume for her next birthday, get her a genie costume and some belly dancing lessons. The lessons will improve her fitness, and when she puts on the genie clobber and does a belly dance—hubba hubba!

3. Sex, alcohol and food — a winning combination

The older we get, the more us blokes begin to enjoy the simple pleasures of good company, good food and good alcohol. There's nothing better than a beer and BBQ, or a bourbon and a burger. We're always up for a chat, a curry and a cab sav, but not always up for sex. Why? Because eating and drinking are fun, laid-back, and involve no performance anxiety—just like sex used to be. So, if we're having a bit of trouble getting our motor running, why not include eating and drinking in our sex life?

Tip for success: Rather than kick back on the sofa with a beer and a pizza, take your partner by the hand and walk her to the bedroom (careful not to spill the beer!), then climb into bed and pour the brew all over her. Throw a couple of slices of pizza onto her midriff and then go to work. Lick the beer off her body and eat the olives out of her belly button—make sure you leave a few slices on the pillow next to her head so you can take a bite or two at the business end of your love-making.

4. Take a visit to the local adult shop

There are many advantages to visiting the local adult shop—we keep our finger on the pulse of what's happening in the world of sex and we can purchase a multitude of gadgets and gizmos for mutual enjoyment with our partners. But by far the biggest advantage is that we can grab a couple of products designed especially for the missus: products that we can use on those nights when we're knackered; that we can pull out from underneath the bed and hand to the missus and say, "Here, baby, I bought you something—go crazy," before rolling over to get a peaceful night's sleep. Everyone's a winner.

Tip for success: Why not take your partner with you when you next visit the local adult shop. She'll love your adventurous spirit; it'll be like your both 18 again, and think of the fun you'll have when you get home and test drive the goodies. Oooh-yeah!

When you're in the mood and she's not

On those rare occasions us men in long-term relationships find the energy for a bit of slap 'n tickle, there's nothing worse than discovering the missus is not interested. Women have the same everyday stresses that us blokes do—work, kids and so on. Plus, they have certain biological stresses that us blokes don't have. If it's the latter that's causing her lack of interest, then we should leave the poor lady alone and look after ourselves. But if it's general tiredness and disinterest, how then do we get her in the mood?

Nowadays, it's not just a case of giving our partners a bit of a rub on the back and a "You up for it, honey?" before throwing the leg over. Nup, women expect a lot more rubbing, tickling, licking, sucking and massaging to get them in the mood. The problem for us blokes, however, is that women are like the cockpit of a Jumbo—there are buttons, knobs, dials, levers and gauges nearly everywhere we look. It's almost like we need eight hands to hit on the combination that will unleash the thrusters and allow the bugger to take off.

As with nearly everything in life, the best answers to complex problems are always the simple ones. Forget all that rubbing, licking and massaging stuff—we'll expend a lot of energy and our partners are still likely to tell us to keep our hands to ourselves. The simple answer is 'champers'—the ultimate leg-opener.

Too easy to be true, I hear you say. Not really. The French invented champagne, and we all know the French don't do much without thinking about how it can get them laid (Pepe le Pew is a prime example). There's something about champers that sets off a woman's erogenous zones like a spark sets off a keg of gunpowder (but don't give her too much, otherwise she's liable to fall asleep or puke). And the great thing about champers is the cheap stuff works just as well as the expensive stuff. She'll loosen up after one glass; after two glasses—giddy-up!

Tip for success: Buy yourself a bottle of champagne on the way home from work, ask her how her day has been and then be prepared to listen. If she's stressed, tell her everything will be fine and then tell her you love her so much that you feel like celebrating. Pop open the champers and get ready to have your clothes ripped off. Nothing will put scratches on your back quicker than this stuff.

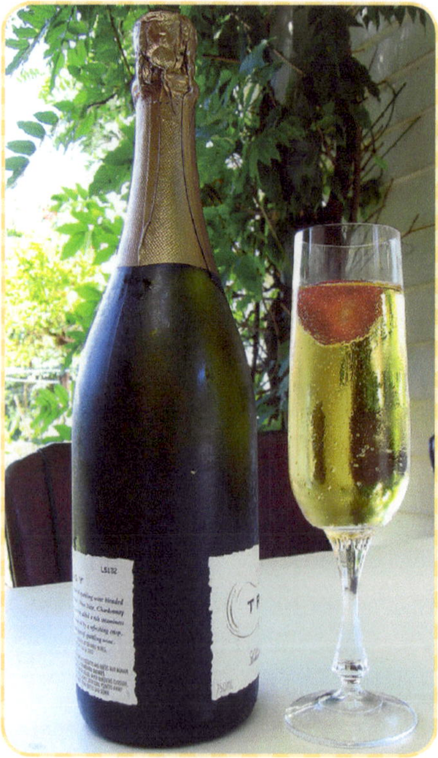

The ultimate leg-opener.

Part 5 — Summary and conclusions

Just because the world is changing, just because women have changed, does it mean that us men must change our very essence to be successful in our long-term relationships? No! Because if we change our essence we lose our identity, and our relationships are then doomed to failure. Rather than change, we should adapt. If we use a few of the techniques described in Part 5 then we too can keep the missus satisfied and become fat and happy.

PART VI

Looking good, feeling great, living well

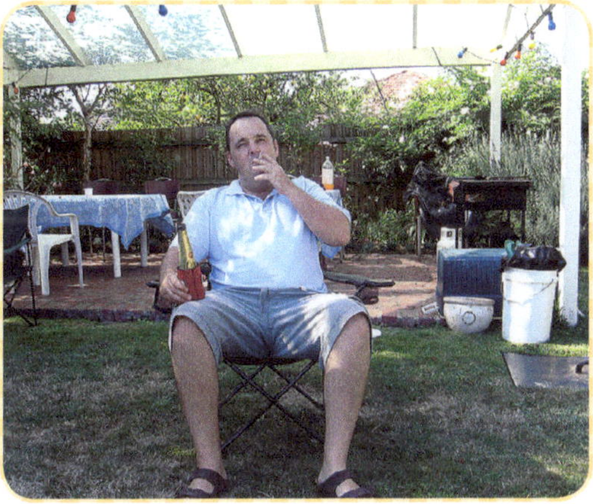

Introduction

Most of us blokes go through stages in our lives when, for one reason or another, we're just not at our best. It may be that the stresses of modern life have gotten the better of us and we've forgotten how to be happy and look after ourselves. Or we're settled in a long-term relationship and we no longer feel the need to impress.

There is nothing wrong with carrying a few extra pounds and spending most of our time bearded-up, unkempt and uncombed, as long as we're secure in who we are and we're happy and healthy. The problems occur when letting ourselves go means that we struggle to spend quality time with the significant others in our lives; when we can't kick a ball around with the kids without the help of an oxygen mask; when the girlfriend is embarrassed to take us along to her end-of-year work function because we look and smell like a hobo.

When we look good and feel great it rubs off on those around us, and our world becomes a better place. And we don't need to pay a fortune for designer clothes, personal trainers or life coaches to get results.

The living well pie

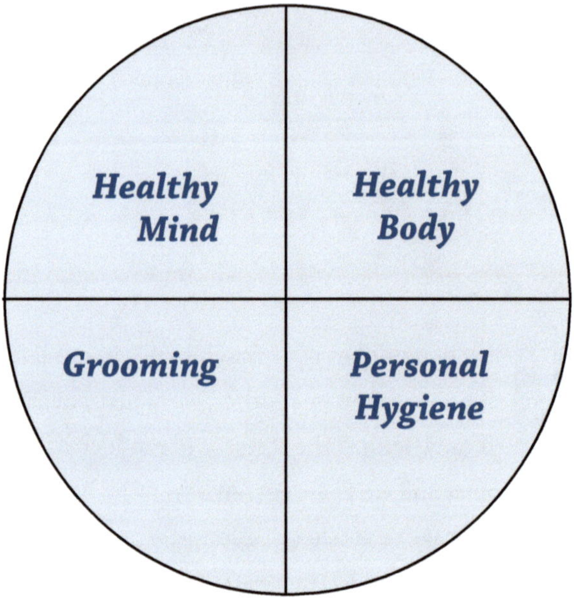

Now let us take a look at each piece of the pie in turn.

Chapter 30 Grooming

When it comes to grooming, there's no need for us men to spend hours in the bathroom pouting and preening ourselves like puffed-up peacocks. We just have to cover the basics.

Hair

On our head

Hair products and expensive styling are all the rage these days. And yes, unfortunately, women do appreciate men who make an effort. But if we don't have the money or we couldn't be bothered, then never discount the good ol' skinhead crew cut—especially if you're thinning on top, as it's a far better option than the ponytail or comb-over. The skinhead is lice and dandruff proof. It's neat, tidy, low maintenance, and it will give us that bad-boy look the chicks really dig. And best of all, we can do it ourselves (or get the missus to do it) with a pair of $10 clippers. How good is that? The shave is the rave.

On the rest of our body

Body hair may have been big in the 70s but it's definitely not the go these days. Hairy men often reassure themselves with the knowledge that body hair is a sign of virility and potency, but it's no good looking like the missing link when the womenfolk run for the hills every time we whip off our shirts. No doubt there are the odd exceptions amongst the opposite sex that buck the trend, and who don't mind their men looking like Chewbacca, but in general they prefer the cleanskin look.

Blokes in long-term relationships may scoff at getting plucked, claiming their partners are used to their hirsute masculinity, but there are certain advantages in doing a bit of deforestation work. Now I'm not advocating blokes waste valuable time every day plucking out every rogue hair that sprouts its ugly head. But every now and again, instead of buying our partners flowers or diamonds for that special occasion, why not surprise them and 'shave down'. Trust me, they'll love it; they'll appreciate not having to furrow through the undergrowth just to find some skin, and all of a sudden they'll start kissing us in places they've never kissed us before, because it will no longer feel like they're kissing a Persian rug.

If we're single and we've got a forest growing out of our nose and ears, and our backs and arses are fire risks, then we've no choice but to get some clearing work done or risk being continually bypassed on the singles' circuit.

> ***Tip for success:*** Whatever you do, don't try hair removal at home. Go to a professional—someone you can trust, someone with expertise and good referrals.

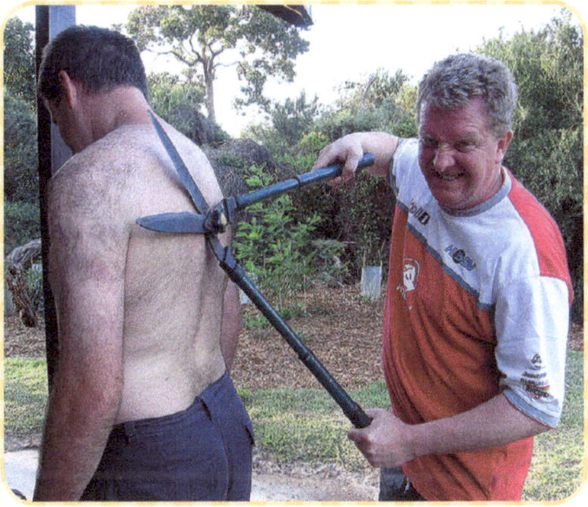

I can highly recommend Big Joe's House of Hair Removal; it's a little backyard operation, but the man knows what he's doing. Big Joe's speciality is the 'Combine Harvester' — especially good for really hairy men.

Smelling good

Nothing will put a woman off quicker than foul body odours, whether they be the foot, underarm, garlic breath or the eight-hour-sitting-at-your-desk-farting type. Smelling like you've just jumped into a river of Brut is a no-no as well. I'm sure we all brush our teeth and shower regularly, but there are some other precautions on top of our basic hygiene routine that we can practice to make sure we always come up smelling like roses.

Feet

Out of sight, out of mind. Most of us don't pay enough attention to our feet because we can't see them in the shower, or because we can't bend over and get to them without slipping and falling bum-over-tit in the process. However, there is an easy way to make sure our feet don't reek, and it involves tomatoes. Yep, tomato juice is about the only thing that can neutralise a skunk's stink, and for a lot of us blokes, the stench of our feet would put a skunk to shame.

Arse

The arse is another trouble-spot for us blokes. Most of us spend the majority of the day sitting on it but only 30 seconds cleaning and deodorising it. The lack of a specific product to target the rectal region hasn't helped our cause; I mean, we have aftershaves, body washes, mouth fresheners, underarm deodorants, all-over deodorants, but nothing—nothing—that targets the bum-hole (the first person to invent an arse-spray will be an instant millionaire!). The only way for us fellas to ensure our butts don't smell like a boggy marsh is to employ a strict deodorising technique. And here's how to do it:

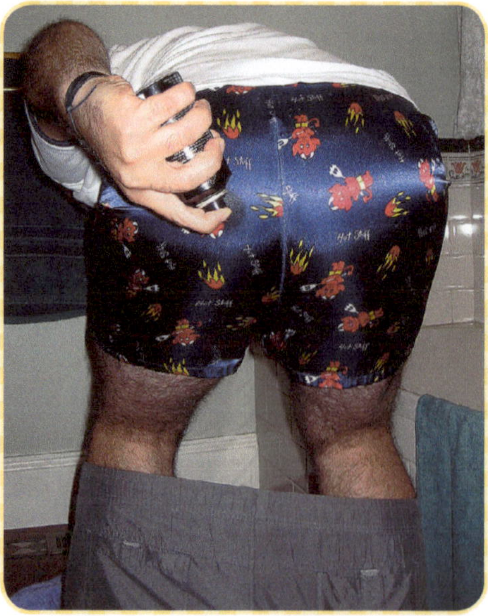

Talc in the jocks and a good deo technique are essential for making sure our bums smell like a rose garden (make sure you tighten the sphincter muscle when applying the spray).

When there's nowhere to shower

Another common mistake that us blokes make when it comes to keeping ourselves smelling nice is to be caught in a situation where we can't freshen up. There's bound to be many occasions—meeting a hot date straight after work, for example—when we don't have access to bathing facilities. And that's exactly the reason it pays to keep an 'odour emergency kit' handy—containing mints, deodorant and talc—in our cars or at our workplaces. The odour emergency kit will allow us to take what I like to term a 'bushman's shower' and consequently avoid 'odour embarrassment'.

Clothes and fashion

Gents, forget about going out and spending thousands on trying to impress the wife or girlfriend. All we need to do when it comes to clothes is remember the following cardinal rules:

Cardinal rule #1: Buy clothes that fit

'Bricklayer's Bum' and 'Visible Gut' are not a good look. Neither are pants, shorts or jeans that are so tight our scrotum is split in two (commonly called 'Fly's Eyes').

Cardinal rule # 2: Fashion is cyclical, so don't throw away your old favourites, because sooner or later they'll be back in fashion

That's right, we keep the old threads no matter how much our partners pressure us to update the wardrobe. Better yet, we keep wearing the old stuff, and sooner or later we'll be back in fashion.

Cardinal rule #3: It's not the clothes, it's the man

Too many of us blokes are brainwashed into thinking we need to have fashion sense to impress the ladies—rubbish! A bloke wearing a cardigan, skivvy and flared jeans can be as attractive to women as a bloke in a Versace suit—it's all about attitude. What's the right attitude? The answer—be happy with who you are, and feel like you have nothing to prove. With this attitude, us blokes could wear a lime-green safari suit for a night out on the town and it wouldn't matter, because some women would find our dagginess appealing. Others may even think we're avant garde or trendy. But all of them will realise that here's a man who's not afraid to be himself. And that, my friends, is worth more than a fashion label.

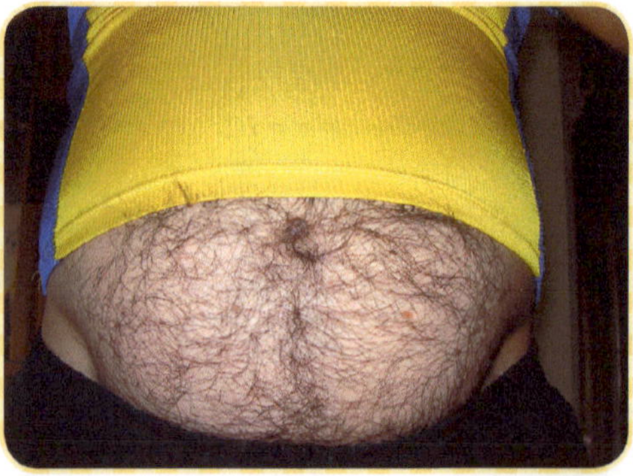

NO!

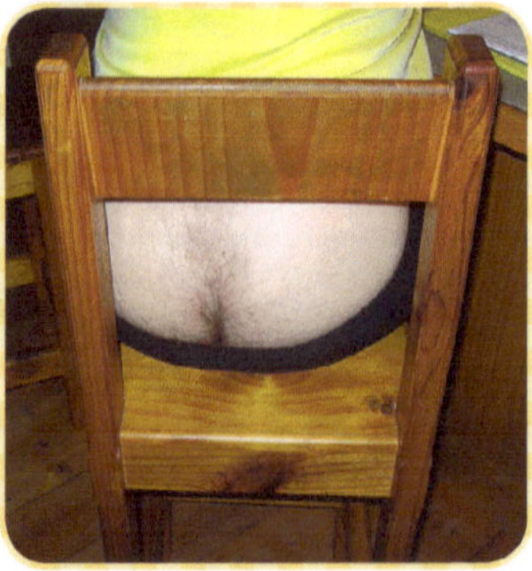

NO!

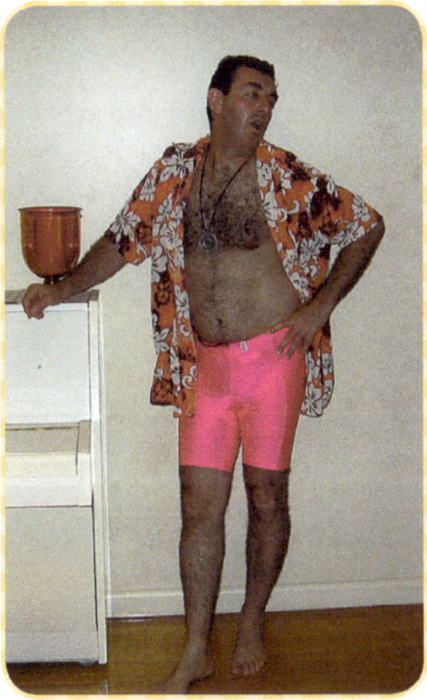

YES!

Teeth and nails

Another huge turnoff for women is bad teeth and long or dirty nails. For the single guy, a lot of hard work can quickly come undone if he cracks a smile that displays a set of teeth only a pirate could love. Just as off-putting as pirate teeth are toenails that could pass for goat hooves, that are tougher than industrial diamonds and are likely to inflict serious injury to partners or bed-mates.

> ***REMEMBER THIS:*** Women rate a great smile right up there in terms of what makes a man attractive. So if we've got nothing else going for us, if we're uglier than all the Rolling Stones put together, then a sure-fire way to keep ourselves in the game is to work at getting a set of choppers that are white and bright enough to guide a ship into shore.

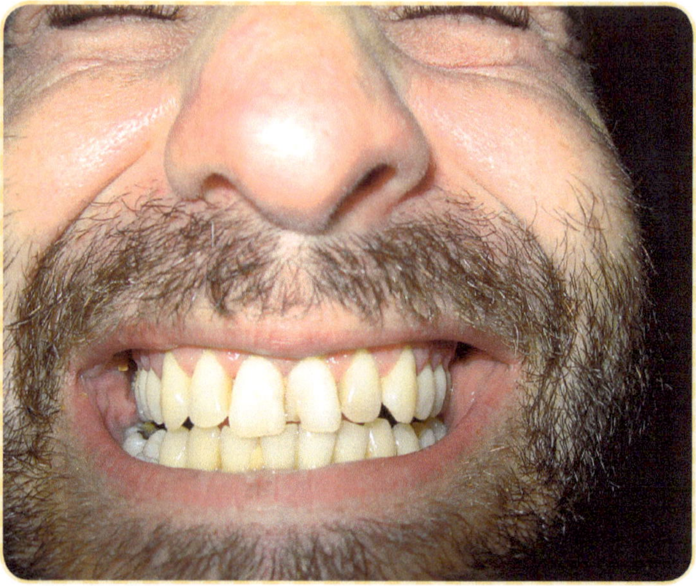

A winning smile will get you a long way.

Chapter 31
Diet and exercise

Say we've had a bumper festive season, or maybe a few too many afternoons drinking beer round the barbeque. Or maybe we're bachelors with no time to cook and a line of credit with the local pizza delivery joint. Whatever the reason, all of a sudden we find ourselves sporting a second chin and suffering a severe bout of *Fatarsis Beerbellyitus*. Is it time to panic? Not necessarily.

It's okay to be a fatty-boomba

Who says we have to be slim, taut and terrific to be happy and healthy? There's nothing wrong with having a 'one-pack' and a set of love handles that spill over our beltline like a well-cooked soufflé spills over its baking dish. Most of us, at some point in our lives, let ourselves go. It happens; it's natural. For the majority, it happens as soon as we get hitched and settle into life with the wife, kids and all the trimmings. But whether we're in a relationship or single, we can be perfectly happy carrying a bit of excess baggage as long as we're secure in our identity and happy on the inside. As long as the pot belly is not causing medical problems or stopping us from enjoying life to the full, then eat, drink and be merry, and who gives a stuff what others think.

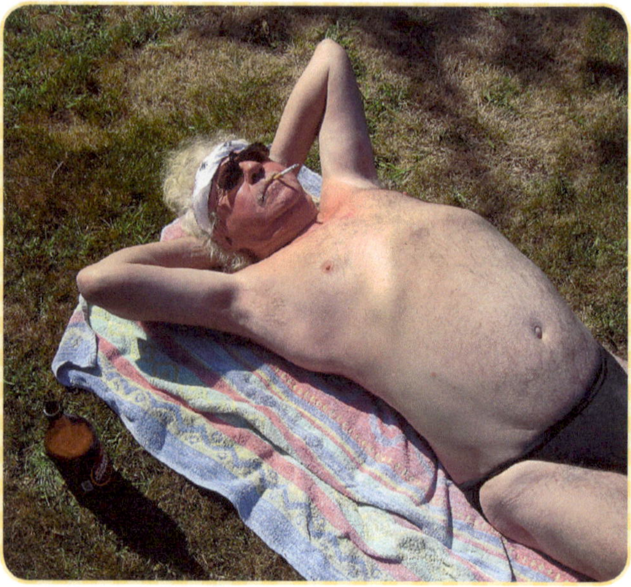

Neighbour Dave — proudly showing off his one-pack.

I wouldn't mind getting back into shape

If our weight and health are stopping us from enjoying life, then it's time we do something about it; but we mustn't be sucked in by miracle cures. Men, by nature, are always looking for the quick fix, and there's thousands of scam-merchants out there pedalling potions, tablets, surgical procedures, and so on and so forth, which promise the world but deliver zip. So remember—DON'T GET SUCKED IN BY MIRACLE CURES!

The other thing we should keep in mind is that getting back into shape doesn't mean just shedding a few pounds. Skinny blokes with bad diets can be just as unhealthy as fat blokes with bad diets. Factors such as cholesterol intake and blood pressure need to be taken into account.

Fellas, there are no 'magic bullets' to getting back into shape. It requires a diet and exercise program that targets all aspects of our health, not just weight. And it requires effort and a willingness to stick to a plan. Does that mean we have to dodge the deep-fried section at Mr Fong's Chinese buffet or count every pea that goes in our gob?—NO! The good news is that we can pretty much eat anything we want as long as we get the essential nutrients we need and pull our fingers out and exercise.

Exercise

"Exercise—that old chestnut. Sounds like too much hard work and I'm too unfit." Rubbish. Just because we have ourselves a set of man-boobs and getting off the couch leaves us short of breath doesn't mean we can't exercise. Trust me, dieting alone won't get us back into shape. Why? Because us blokes are glutinous creatures who, despite our best intentions, can't help eating everything that's put in front of us.

Exercising doesn't mean running a marathon every second day; nor does it mean forking out good money on a gym membership or the latest whiz-bang exercise machine that we'll only ever use once. The trick with exercise is to do something we enjoy; something that will provide a total body workout; something that can be a social event as well as a fat burning one. Choosing an activity that fits these criteria is the only way to guarantee we do it regularly.

Top 5 exercises for those wanting to get back into shape

1. Golf—can't beat it; it's social and it gets us out of the house and into shape, providing we don't do it with a motorised golf cart stocked full of beer.
2. Sex—what a way to burn them calories.
3. Walking—unlikely to injure ourselves and good for us.
4. Dance classes—all the rage, great workout for the body as well as the eyes, and a great way to meet women if we're single.
5. Swimming/dog paddling—easy on the joints and gets us clean as well.

Diet

Let's make no bones about it—most of us blokes have diets guaranteed to clog whole sewer systems let alone arteries. When we're bachelors living alone or sharing, it's often much easier to pick up the phone and order in or hit the drive-thru rather than waste valuable time shopping and preparing food. And when it's the wife's night off, what man in his right mind could be stuffed preparing a dinner when a bucket of chicken will do the job nicely? Grabbing a meat pie and chips from the canteen at work is much more tempting than a salad sanger. And who wants water or juice when we can drink beer or something fizzy and full of sugar?

For most blokes, the problem isn't eating too much, it's eating too much of one thing (typically fried stuff, fast foods or processed foods) that can lead to health issues. Am I saying we need to give up all the foods we love? Hell no! Eating is one of life's joys. Rather than take the 'cut out' approach to dieting, I prefer the 'supplement' approach. In other words, we eat what we like but we make sure we add the essential vitamins and minerals our bodies need.

There are supplements on the market for every health concern known to man—multivitamin tablets for vitamin deficiency, fibre for constipation, fish oil for cholesterol concerns, and so on. But to avoid us blokes having to take a fistful of tablets and powders to supplement our crappy diets, I have developed a recipe that combines all the most beneficial active ingredients in one easy-to-swallow 'wunderdrink' which I call 'Miracle Man Juice'. And providing we drink one glass per day and do some exercise, why not have pizza seven days a week, morning, noon and night. Miracles happen.

Miracle Man Juice — ingredients

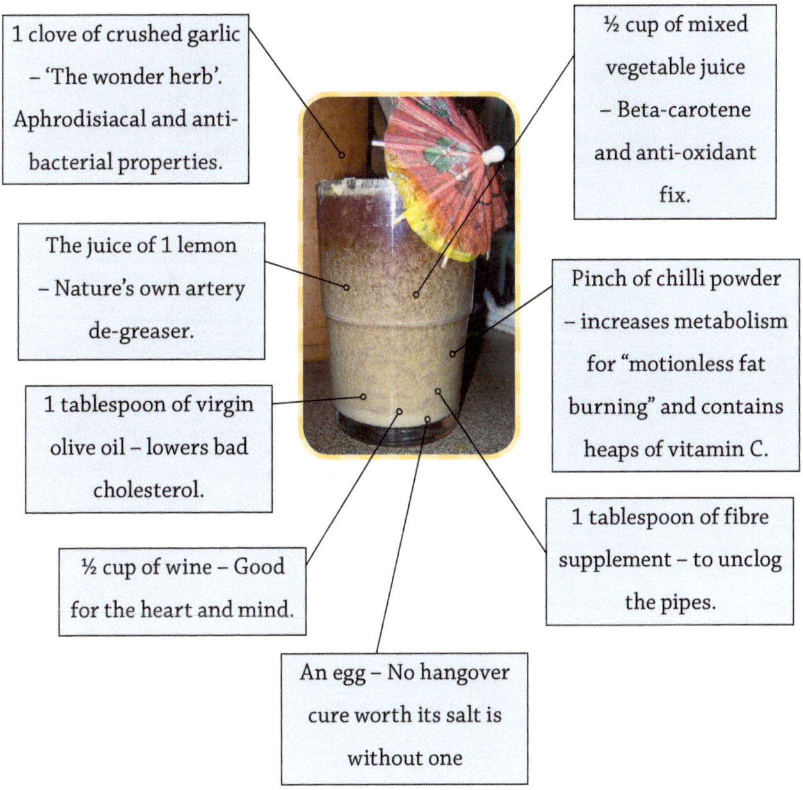
1 clove of crushed garlic – 'The wonder herb'. Aphrodisiacal and anti-bacterial properties.
½ cup of mixed vegetable juice – Beta-carotene and anti-oxidant fix.
The juice of 1 lemon – Nature's own artery de-greaser.
Pinch of chilli powder – increases metabolism for "motionless fat burning" and contains heaps of vitamin C.
1 tablespoon of virgin olive oil – lowers bad cholesterol.
1 tablespoon of fibre supplement – to unclog the pipes.
½ cup of wine – Good for the heart and mind.
An egg – No hangover cure worth its salt is without one

Handy hint: Miracle Man Juice also works well on stubborn driveway oil stains, and as a paint stripper.

Miracle Man Juice, the miracle magic bullet quick fix that us men have been waiting for. If you need proof, take one look at neighbour Dave flexing his muscles after downing a glass of the stuff — fit as a mallee bull, could chew iron. Onya, champ!

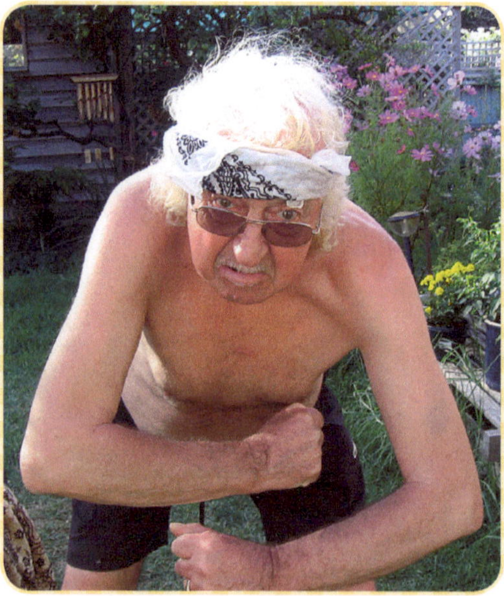

Chapter 32
A healthy mind

Modern day society is full of stressors for us men: work pressures, family worries, money concerns, body image, relationships—the list goes on. Given our egos, most of us blokes find it hard to admit that we're under stress; as a result, we go about our business trying to cope until one day the stress levels get the better of us and we fall in a heap. If we've forgotten how to enjoy ourselves, if minor things tick us off, if our mind races from one worry to the next, then we're stressed and we need to do something about it.

So how do we get that stress circuit-breaker? Yoga, Tai-Chi and the thousands of other meditation techniques do work, but most of us blokes don't want to risk our nuts popping out of our shorts while we try our best to put one foot behind our ear—it's not a good look and it's hard work. Plus, there are time and cost factors that put men off signing up to classes. There are easier, more economical and enjoyable ways to relieve stress. The trick is to meditate without even knowing you're meditating.

It's all about focusing the mind

The basic principle of meditation is to focus the mind and clear it of all the other extra stressful stuff. If we're mildly stressed, then a good session in front of the TV will usually do the trick. If the stress levels are higher, then retreating to our own 'personal space area' of the house with a good bottle of red and a few favourite CDs is sure to work wonders. But if the stress levels are hardcore, then we need to clear the mind and focus—and here's how we do it:

Fishing

A fantastic stress reliever. All the setting up, rigging and casting focuses the mind and clears it out, which enables us to concentrate on other things, such as the great outdoors—the sounds, the smells and the sights. Even if we don't catch anything, we'll feel refreshed after an afternoon on the pier.

> ***Tip for success:*** Results are best when you go alone, but you can still reap the benefits if you go with a car load of mates; because unlike women, men can be with their mates and still be in their own little world, with the only sound to pass between them being that of two cans opening simultaneously at regular intervals.

Gardening

Same deal as with fishing, although best to leave the mates out of this one unless we want constant advice on how to do things better. Getting our hands dirty, the smell of loam and the physical exertion will all help clear the mind. Plus, after a day's gardening, guaranteed we'll have a crook back and pains all over—and pain is another great way to focus the mind and make us forget everything else.

Music

If we're single and living in a small pad with no garden, and fishing sounds like a waste of valuable time, then we can learn to play a musical instrument. Learning to play an instrument requires absolute concentration, and will focus our mind on the task at hand. But for goodness sakes, we must make sure we choose an instrument that suits—bagpipes in a block of flats is more likely to get us arrested than relieve our stress.

Projects

My old man used to build stuff all the time, only to knock his creations down months later and start again on something new. Why? Stress relief. Banging, chopping, sawing, cutting—all mind-focusers. There's something inherently satisfying in taking to a chunk of wood with a giant axe or firing up the acetylene torch with enough punch to melt a gold ingot. Whether it be rebuilding a car, brewing homemade beer, knocking together an outdoor setting or engineering the mother of all barbeques, having a project to work on is a great way to relieve stress.

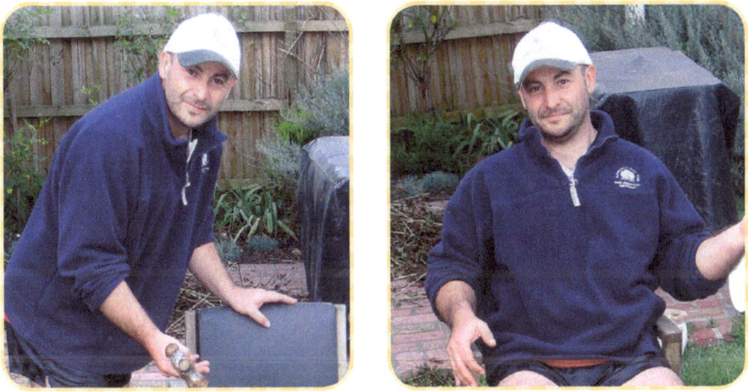

The author, proud of his restoration of an old chair.

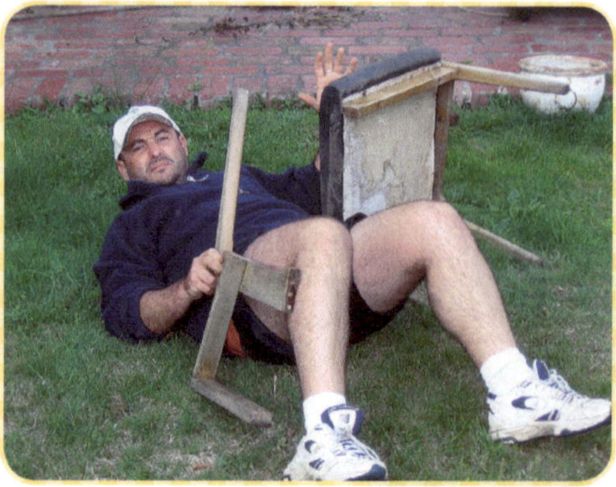

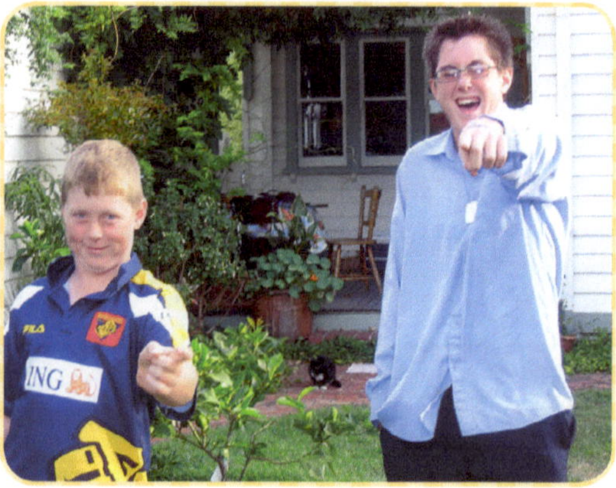

Projects are such a great stress reliever!

Chapter 33
First aid for common male ailments

These days the cost of medicine is astronomical, and if we're really sick then we don't have much choice but to cough up the cash. However, there are every-day ailments that afflict us men which could be taken care of with some good old-fashioned home-grown remedies. For thousands of years, we humans have managed without the wonders of modern medicine by making use of the healing properties found in herbs and plants. Unfortunately, a lot of this knowledge has been lost through the generations. I have made it my mission to rediscover it.

After months of web surfing, scouring information on the herb lore wisdom of ancient civilisations (and some not so ancient), I have gathered together a collection of cures that are readily available around the house; cures for ailments that are more nuisance than nasty but nevertheless end up costing us a packet.

Itchy scrote

Description
A fungal condition that affects the nut-sack, causing an extremely annoying irritation that makes us men want to regularly reach down and give the 'boys' a good scratching.

Cure
Garlic—nature's own wonder herb. Reputed anti-fungal and anti-bacterial properties. A poultice of crushed garlic regularly applied to the ghoolie-bag will clear up that nasty itchy scrote in no time.

Athlete's foot

Description
Fungal infection from the same family as itchy scrote. Ironically named, as most people that suffer from the condition are allergic to exercise. Usually occurs between the toes.

Cure
Soaking our socks in vinegar works well. So too does taking a leak on our feet (we DO NOT do this in the shower if we value our lives, because if the missus catches us—yikes!)

Flatulence

Description
Excess wind as a result of consuming foods (baked beans, curries, cruciferous vegetables) that when digested cause an excess level of gas to be produced in our system.

Cure

Charcoal is the answer, and charcoal tablets are readily available. Otherwise we can suck on a briquette or chew on some charred wood left over from the last night's BBQ or log fire.

Shagger's back

Description

Usually occurs as a result of an overestimation of our ability and flexibility when we're 'on the job' executing a technically challenging shag move. Once sustained, easily aggravated by normal everyday activities such as lying on the couch for prolonged periods of time. Symptoms include lower back pain and inflammation.

Cure

For severe cases we ice the affected area, and keep icing it at hourly intervals for a couple of days. When the inflammation has gone down we can try some gentle massage with eucalyptus oil. If we have a wife and kids, then we lay on our back on a hard floor and get the kids to take our feet, pulling in one direction, while the wife takes our arms and pulls in the opposite direction, until we hear a crack or pop. If we're single, we get a couple of mates to do the same thing the next time we're legless.

Haemorrhoids

Description

These little nasties make us blokes feel like we're clutching a couple of cherry tomatoes between our arse cheeks. They can be extremely uncomfortable. Caused by pressure on the blood vessels around, and in, the bum-hole—typically from trying to strangle out a turd that's so hard it clinks all the way down the s-bend.

Cure

Fibre in the diet will help in prevention. While afflicted, we could try a warm salty bath to reduce the swelling. If we haven't got a bath then we go wash our arse in the ocean: the sea water will work wonders.

Part 6 — Summary and conclusions

Guys, we don't have to become gym-junkies or Yoga masters to live well. We don't have to spend heaps of time shopping for clothes or primping and preening. All that's required is a sensible approach to diet and exercise, as well as a bit of time-out every now and again. And when it comes to grooming and fashion, we shouldn't let others dictate what we have to wear. If we have the right attitude, then we can wear just about anything and still impress the hell out of our partners and girlfriends. And in any case, those that love us will realise it's the man they love, not the clothes, and will forgive us our occasional fashion transgressions.

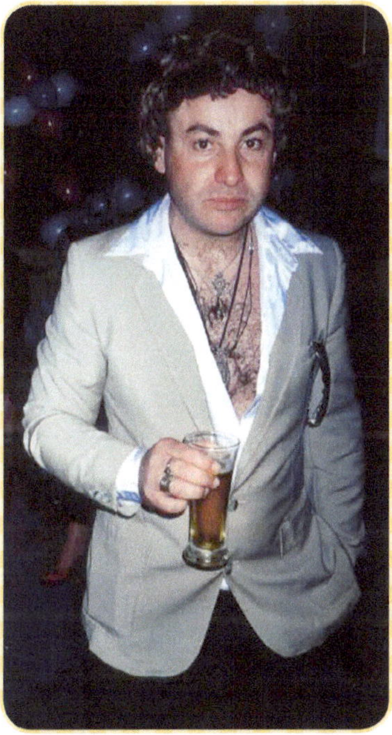

Dressed to impress — work it, baby, work it!

PART VII

A user's guide to alcohol

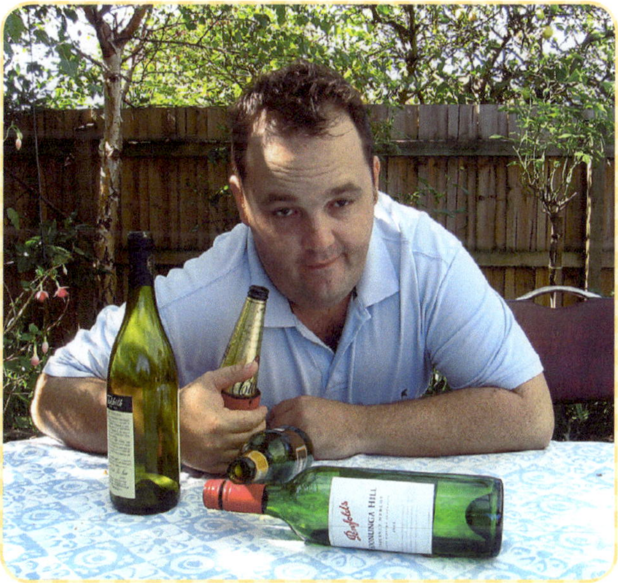

Chapter 34
Know your poison

"He was a wise man who invented beer."
(Source: Plato)

For many of us, drinking alcohol is a rite of passage in our youth and a big part of the social fabric that makes up our lives as we get older. Sure, these days there are lots of other social drugs available to the consumer, but alcohol is still the most commonly used—and abused. And that's why men of all ages need to know their way around booze.

There are tons of books, videos and courses out there that can teach us men lots about the different types of alcoholic beverages available, about how to appreciate them, even how to make them. But a lot of this information is useless to the everyday social drinker—especially those just reaching drinking age. More than anything, what us blokes need to know is how to enjoy alcohol and stay out of trouble, because there's a lot more to grog then just drinking the stuff.

Not all alcohol is the same

There is an old saying amongst pubgoers that goes something like: "Don't matter what you're drinking because it all has the same effect." Wrong! Different types of alcohol affect us in different ways. Basically, there are three types of alcoholic beverages:

1. **Softcore (2% — 20% alcohol by volume)**
   This category includes drinks such as beer, cider, spritzers, punch and wine, which if drunk responsibly will gently creep up on us and slowly loosen our inhibitions, giving us a mellow buzz. Ideal for social occasions such as dinners or BBQs, but over-consumption can result in behaviours such as breaking out the karaoke machine or flirting with a mate's wife.

2. **Midcore (20% — 40% alcohol by volume)**
   This category includes all your classic spirits: scotch, bourbon, whiskey, vodka, as well as liqueurs and fortified wines. Midcore drinks hit harder and faster than their softcore counterparts. A couple of these babies can help relax us and take the edge off a particularly stressful day or occasion. But how many of us stop at a couple? Not many. Plus, we mix these drinks with all kinds of mixers that can change the character of the drink and lend it an energetic or aggressive buzz, resulting in behaviours such as dusting off the Black Sabbath and Deep Purple records and giving the old air guitar a good workout, or grabbing our best mate in a headlock and shouting "I luv ya, brother!" before hitting the dance floor in a manner that suggests we've just been shot with a Taser gun.

3. Hardcore (40%+ alcohol by volume)

We're talking Grappa, overproof spirits, rocket-fuel and the like. One shot of these bad-boys and we'll feel like we've swallowed a ball of molten lava. Typically drunk at bucks' nights. When drinking this stuff there's not much conversation involved; instead, after each shot there is a lot of loud exhaling, grunting, high-fiving, eye bulging and yelling. In fact, most partakers of hardcore alcohol end up acting like berserk Vikings preparing for war. BEWARE—hardcore strength drinks don't creep up on us, they hit us like freight trains. Drink too many too quickly and we'll be yelling and beating our chests one moment, then reduced to incoherent, shambling zombies the next—and that's only if we're lucky. If we're unlucky, we'll end up comatose and at the mercy of our mates.

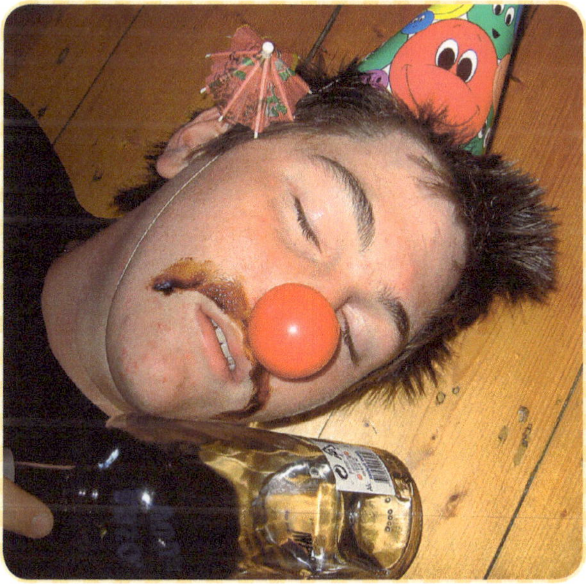

Chapter 35
Alcohol and status

There is a school of thought that suggests we can tell the character of a man by what he drinks. There are a lot of posers out there drinking certain types of alcohol, not because they enjoy it but because they believe drinking the stuff elevates them into a higher class. These types of guys can easily be classified into the following groups:

The weekend wine expert

I'm sure we've all come across one or two of these fellows around the traps. The type of gent who rocks up to a dinner with friends brandishing a swish bottle of plonk, telling everyone how much it cost before launching into a lecture on palette and vintage. If someone dares ask for a taste, this dude reacts with shock before advising all and sundry that this quality of wine needs time to 'breathe'. Give me a break.

The beer racist

This guy turns his nose up at local beers, preferring to stick to the European varieties in the belief that drinking the imported stuff somehow elevates his status above the everyday rank and file. The type of guy who only enters a shout if everyone else is prepared to buy him the expensive gear. He also thinks anyone drinking beer from a tap or a keg is uncouth.

The young wannabees

Probably the biggest posers of all. The type of guys who join exclusive clubs; the type that take every opportunity to associate themselves with the perceived 'upper crust' in the hope of climbing the social ladder. Will not drink anything that isn't black label, blue label, French, VSOP or premium, and rarely associate with anyone that doesn't do the same.

The culture vulture

The type who tries to set himself up as worldly and cultured by demonstrating a knowledge of international alcoholic beverage types and brands. Often 'name drops' obscure alcoholic varieties in order to impress—something along the lines of, "I quite enjoy a Pernod before my meal; I discovered it whilst in the south of France." The more these guys drink, and the more the other guests ignore them, the more outlandish their stories become: "You call that vodka? Now when I was trekking across the Russian steppe, chased by a pack of rabid Siberian huskies, I took shelter in a nearby inn where I was served a vodka brewed on special request by none other than Rasputin himself." Sad, isn't it? Very sad.

Drink for enjoyment and not for status

Just because we rock up to a restaurant to meet the wife's new boss with a bottle of 12-buck-chuck or a slab of local beers doesn't mean we're any less of a man than the bloke walking in with the bottle of Grange or a six-pack of Grolsch. Just because our idea of an after-dinner palette cleanser is necking another can of beer, while others partake in a cognac or single-malt scotch, doesn't mean we lack culture. Just because we pop the question with a $10 bot of spumante, as opposed to the Dom Perignon, don't mean we lack class.

At the end of the day, if we're secure in our identity then we drink whatever we like, and those around us will end up respecting us for not trying to be something we're not.

Chapter 36
Traps for young players

The open wallet syndrome

Often, when we've had too much to drink, we suddenly feel the urge to shout every Tom, Dick and Harry at the bar. Or we are overcome with a sudden desire to ditch the beer and basic spirits and hit the cocktails and top-shelf stuff. Just as alcohol loosens up our sexual inhibitions, so too does it loosen up our purse strings.

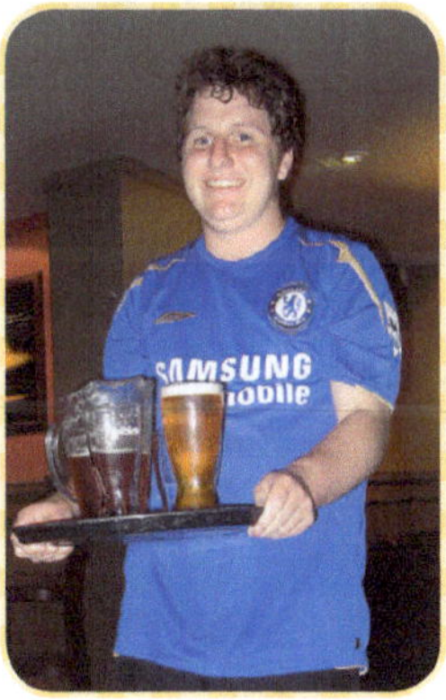

Young Matty is feeling no pain as he celebrates with a few ales after scoring a hat-trick for his soccer club. Overcome by the occasion, he decides to start buying the rounds for the lads.

Factors likely to trigger off the open wallet syndrome are many—a new job, a new girlfriend, celebrating a special occasion or just showing off. This sudden onset of generosity and big spending will most likely make us the most popular guy in the pub, but the impact on our finances can be devastating.

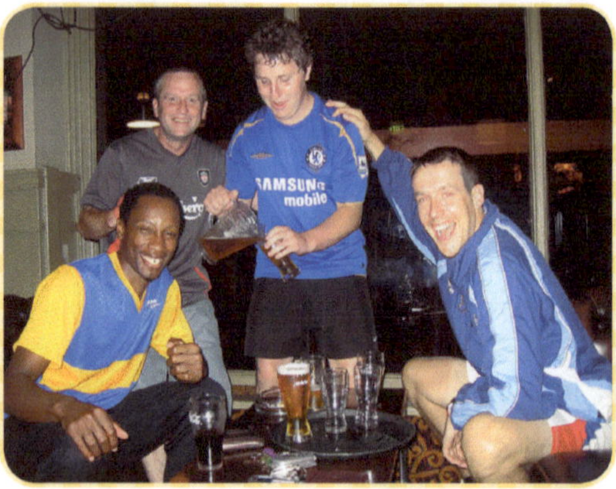

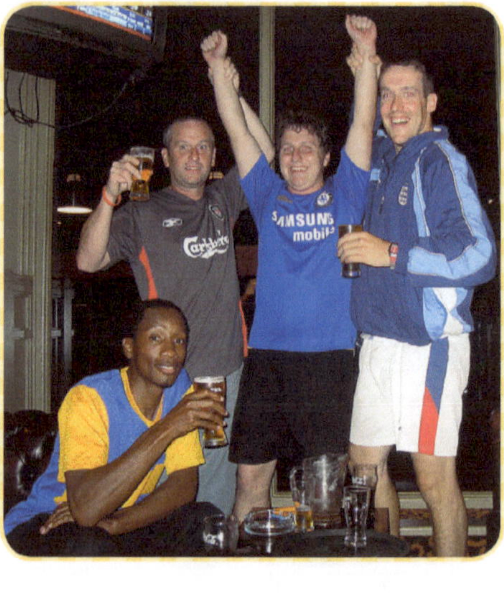

Young Matty buying yet another round and becoming the most popular bloke in the pub.

The bottom line is, we don't shout anyone who is unlikely to shout us back, and we resist the temptation to buy anything with a multicoloured paper umbrella and a few chunks of fruit sticking out of the top of the glass.

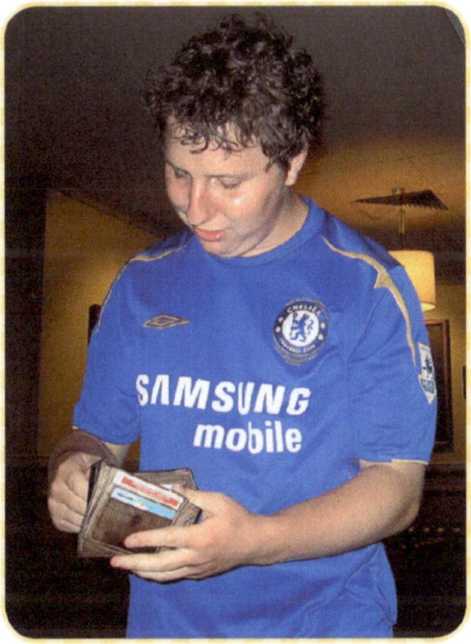

The lads have all gone home, leaving Matty alone with his empty wallet—yet another victim of the open wallet syndrome. Remember, Matty—he who shouts last, laughs loudest!

Drinks that will get us into trouble

There are certain drinks on the market that are more likely than others to land us blokes in hot water. I could mention many here—Depth Charges, Long Island iced teas, sangria (a Spanish drink made from fermented fruit that infuses the drinker with an unexplained yearning to run in front of stampeding bulls) and vodka mixed with caffeine-based energy drinks, just to name a few. But I will instead focus on the most notorious.

1. Tequila

Also known as *Te-kill-ya* or Mexican fire-water. This stuff is the devil's own brew. It's made from cacti—which we all know are full of pricks, and that's exactly what we turn into if we drink too much of the stuff. Sooner or later in our drinking careers we'll be involved in a round of 'slammers', and my advice is to stop at two. One or two can set us up for a good night; any more than that and for five minutes we'll feel like we could catch a lightning bolt between our teeth, but sooner or later it will catch up with us, and when it does it's lights out, good-night.

2. Rum

"If you drink rum and don't fight, then you're a fucking coward."
(Source: Unknown, probably a sailor)

The favoured drink of sailors, rough-heads and brawlers. There's something about this world famous beverage that brings out the animal in us blokes. Three or four glasses of this stuff and even the most mild-mannered office accountant is likely to go the first bloke who looks at him sideways.

Tip for success: If you plan on drinking rum, or hanging around with people who drink rum, you had better learn how to handle yourself.

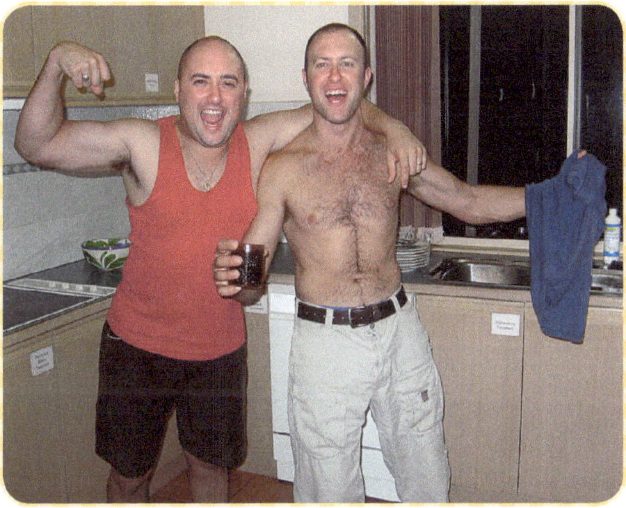

A few Te-kill-ya shots and a couple of rums and the brothers Colasante are ready to take on the world!

Skulling, slamming and chugging

Some men fight to prove their manhood, others play sport or drive fast cars. Then there are those who like to prove their manhood by downing their drinks in a single gulp. Unfortunately, it's not enough for these raving lunatics to write themselves off, they have to take others down with them. Generally, these blokes skull one drink after the other in quick succession, laugh in the face of danger (and health risks), and challenge everyone around them to do the same. Those who don't take up the challenge are likely to be on the end of some serious taunts—"weak as piss", "Nancy-boys", and so on and so forth.

DO NOT SUCCUMB TO PEER PRESSURE. Our guts are not designed to take on large quantities of liquid quickly, and skull-ing our drinks will inevitably end up in us performing the 'evil

Exorcist puke' (a spasm of the gut that comes on violently and unexpectedly, projecting the contents of our stomachs out of our mouths in a single stream at high velocity), which can be very embarrassing for the puker, and anyone else who happens to cop a bit of friendly-fire.

Letting the excitement and anticipation of a night out get the better of us

Especially relevant for men in long-term relationships, and those who have settled into a family routine and have forgotten what the inside of a pub looks like. On the rare occasion that these men do get the 'call-up' for a night out on the town with the lads—and they are able to secure a leave pass from their better halves—they tend to get so excited about reliving their long-lost glory days that they literally burst out of the cab and knock down the door of the pub in their rush to get stuck into it. Sure, they may give it a good nudge for an hour or two—drinking like there's no tomorrow, chatting up girls half-their age and ridiculing the young blokes for being wimps—but the end result is usually a sad old man unlikely to see the other side of 10 pm before falling fast asleep face-down in his bowl of chips.

Arriving 'cold'

There's nothing worse than rocking up to a big do stone cold sober, only to find that everyone else is lagered to the hilt. When we're sober, drunk people seem to speak a different language; in fact they may as well be from another planet. When we arrive cold, everyone will ply us with drinks to try and get us up to speed, and we're bound to drink them quickly in order to catch up—DANGER!

The big event syndrome and piss fitness

Throughout the course of a year we're likely to be invited to a huge bash or two—a wedding, the work Christmas party or a New Year's Eve do, for example. It is at these big events that those who don't normally drink get caught up in the sense of occasion and proceed to hit the bottle full-boar, only to end up making real fools of themselves. Why do they make fools of themselves? Because they're not 'piss fit'.

We wouldn't attempt a marathon without doing a few kilometres on the training track to prepare the body. The same principle applies when it comes to attending a special occasion where the booze will be free-flowing and everyone will be in the mood to party. Piss fitness can only be achieved gradually, over a period of time. So if we know there's a huge occasion on the horizon, then some time before the event we need to begin preparing the body.

> ***Tip for success:*** Let's take the silly season of Christmas/New Year's as a case study. Come December 1st, begin a regimen of at least two beers (or whatever your poison is) every night with dinner. Step it up each day until you're polishing off around 5 or 6 beers a night, and then maintain that level for the week prior to the function. By the time the function comes round you'll be piss fit and unlikely to do something you may regret for the rest of your life.

The 'talking crap' syndrome

We all have one—a mate who gets on the piss and starts talking crap. Why? Because alcohol has this wonderful capability of tapping into previously unused areas of the male brain and unleashing hitherto hidden intellectual powers. An ordinary, everyday type of bloke who's overindulged can all of a sudden become an expert on every topic known to man, with the uncanny ability to draw on facts and figures, and even quote statistics, steadfastly convinced that all the crap coming out of his mouth is undeniable truth. In addition to this, he uncovers a previously unknown creative flair for storytelling, resulting in him enthralling his audience with tales of his sexual exploits, athletic prowess and fighting expertise, all filled with the most intricate of details (even if none of them actually occurred) and recounting them in a manner that would make the world's bestselling fiction writers proud. Fellas, a reputation for 'talking crap' is not something we should aspire to.

Chapter 37
Hangovers

We've all been there. Work Christmas party; free booze; doomed attempts at cracking on to anything in a skirt after four rounds of tequila shots; escorted off the hotel premises by some do-gooder from accounts payable; moon every taxi that doesn't stop before taking a wizz in the hotel fountain, only to loose our balance and fall in. Eventually get home and stumble into bed, only to find the room beginning to spin, causing us to make a frantic beeline for the toilet, where we spend the next few hours paying homage to the porcelain gods before passing out and waking up the next morning with our head still resting on the bowl, feeling like death warmed up.

Unfortunately, hangovers are a part of life; but we can employ a few tactics to make coping with the evil beastie a lot easier. The first part of coping is understanding.

The anatomy of a hangover

Nearly all hangovers have the following elements: furry teeth, death-breath, saliva that could glue bathroom tiles together, dry-cork tongue and a throbbing headache. In more severe cases, complete episodes from the night before will have been erased from our memory. Less severe cases involve periodic flashbacks that can occur spontaneously or when reminded of our exploits by a third party.

In addition to the above symptoms, there are the 'mystery injuries' to deal with—unaccountable sprains, cuts and bruises. Injuries we couldn't feel, or notice sustaining, the night before but begin to hurt like crazy now that we've sobered up.

And to rub salt into the wounds, we'll most likely waste the rest of the following day on the couch—watching TV, moaning and groaning, vowing "never again"—while we desperately wait to feel human again. As soon as we do, the first thing we crave is some artery-clogging deep-fried junk food.

Coping with a hangover

Hangovers are basically caused by dehydration. A heavy night on the turps leeches the body of its store of liquids and its supplies of vitamins and minerals. Forget all the gimmicky stuff on the market claiming to rid us of our hangovers, because hangovers are like the common cold—there is no cure. All we can do is ease the symptoms. But if we do the following, we'll feel better in no time:

- Force ourselves to drink water to flush the system—at least one litre every hour.

- Take a couple of multivitamin pills, not just B-group vitamins.
- Buy some rehydration fluid from the pharmacist (the stuff that contains mineral salts and electrolytes) and drink plenty of it.
- Stay away from spicy or oily foods—just broth or plain rice, thanks very much.
- Take a Panadol thickshake—blend together, in a tall glass, 250ml milk, ice cream, two paracetamol/aspirin tablets, one raw egg and a banana.
- Sleep as much as you can.

Alternatively, ‘hair of the dog’ works wonders.

Chapter 38
Other unwanted by-products of a night out on the turps

Looking after a drunk mate

Every now and again in our socialising careers, one of the lads will have had way too many and will proceed to make a complete arsehole of himself before collapsing in a heap. This usually happens when we're having a great time ourselves, so what do we do in this situation? Ignore him? Disown him?

Among the male fraternity, nothing will earn us more respect than helping out a drunk mate; it's right up there with helping a mate in a fight. Also, keep in mind that it may be us who needs the help one day, so do unto others ... Even if we're getting somewhere with the most beautiful girl in the room, if our mate needs help then we have to put him first (unless she's really, really good-looking, then it's a case of bugger him, he can look after himself). Here are some useful tips on how to help out a drunk mate.

If he's loud and abusive and generally making a pig of himself

We tell him to settle down; if this doesn't work, we punch him in the guts, hard enough to take the wind out of his sails. He won't hold it against us if he understands we did it with the best possible intention—to stop him making a complete dick of himself.

If he's passed out

We carry him out of the venue fireman-style, making sure the ladies see us doing it. While we're carrying him out we say stuff like, "Don't worry, mate, I've got you; I'll look after you." By doing this we're making the most of a bad situation—we're helping a mate and impressing the hell out of the ladies at the same time. Once we get him home, it's time to hose him down, dry him off and put him to bed.

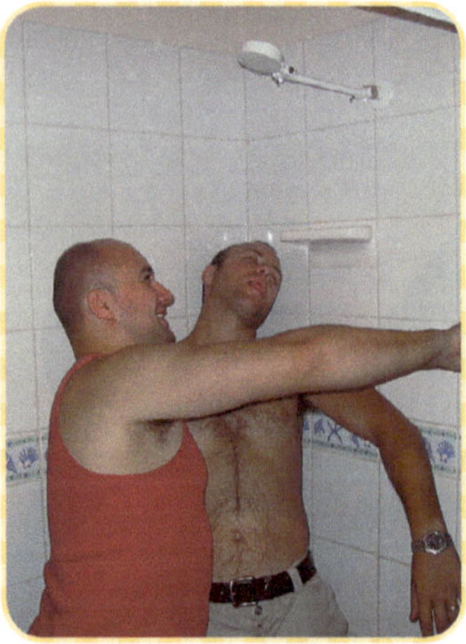

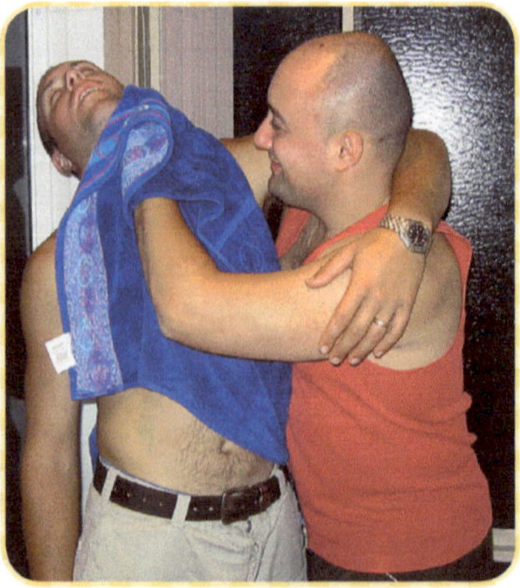

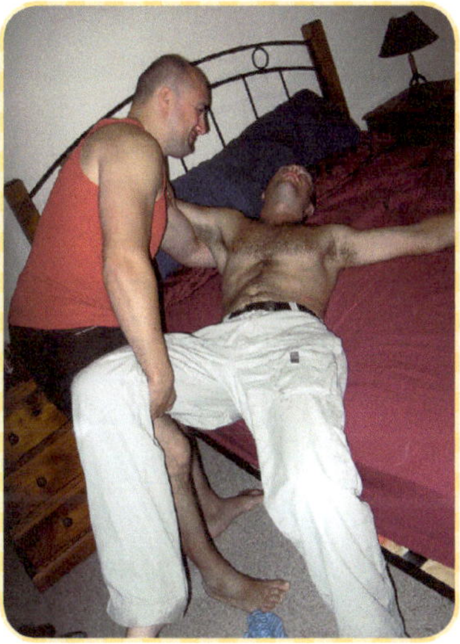

The 'hose-down, dry-off, put-to-bed' combo is the most intimate thing one man can do for another in the heterosexual world — it's the sign of true mateship.

Damage control

Another unwanted by-product of a big night out is the need for damage control. We may not make fools of ourselves every time we go out (and hopefully, with experience, we'll learn to heed the danger signs and keep our mouths shut) but, rest assured, we will make fools of ourselves on the odd occasion.

Damage control is all about being prepared, proactive, creative and quick on our feet. Say we've had a huge night, and now, in the cold harsh light of the morning, we're starting to experience flashbacks that make us cringe at our own stupidity. Rather than sit around and wait for the proverbial to hit the fan, we get up off of our sorry arse, jump on the phone, call up the sister-in-law and explain that it wasn't "What I'd give to see you bend over and touch your toes" that we actually said, but "What I'd give to get rid of this runny nose." Easy—the spark is snuffed out before it becomes a raging inferno.

> ***Tip for success:*** Have a list of excuses handy just in case one of the gals at work bails you up on a Monday morning wanting explanations for your unruly behaviour:
>
> - The medication I was on made me silly.
> - Someone spiked my drink.
> - I hadn't slept for three days and the grog just went to my head.
> - I wasn't actually pinching your bum, I was just trying to pick off some lint.

If we're prepared, proactive, creative and quick on our feet, we'll avoid our fair share of after-party controversy. But if we've been really, really bad boys, then our best hope is to go underground—lay low or take extended leave—until everything blows over.

Too drunk to funk

Alcohol can have a positive effect on our sexual performance by enflaming our desire, giving us increased staying power and making us more adventurous. BUT there's a fine line between the positive and the negative. Too much alcohol and we'll be about as useful as a bike with no wheels—she can sit on our seat and try and ride us but she won't be going anywhere, and neither will we.

The 'heavy pants' syndrome

How many times do us blokes find ourselves having to walk home because we've got no moolah for the cab fare or the train ticket? How many times are our pockets full of change but our wallets empty of cash? How many times have we wondered—as we stumble homewards at some ungodly hour, bogged down by our jean pockets overflowing with coins, jingling and jangling like one of Santa's reindeer—where all our money went?

Us blokes end up spending wads of cash on our nights out because we fail to take into account the miscellaneous expenses, such as the mandatory 3 am kebab, souvlaki, pizza or hot dog. If we want to make sure we have the cab fare at the end of the night then we must have a budget in mind.

> ***Tip for success:*** Your budget should take into account some or all of the following:

- Cab fares/public transport.
- Standard drinks; eg, beer.
- Fancy drinks; eg, spirits and cocktails.
- Shouting mates.
- Buying ladies drinks.
- Coffees.
- Cigars/smokes.
- Chips and nuts.
- End of night junk food, for when you've lucked out with the ladies and decide to compensate by eating the greasiest food you can find.

Handy hint: Keep your cab fare money in a separate pocket, stick to your budget, and leave ATM and credit cards at home. When you run out of drinking money, sponge of some sucker suffering from the open wallet syndrome, or go home.

Chapter 39
The step-by-step guide to handling your drink

So far I've outlined the traps we can fall into where alcohol is concerned, and the unwanted by-products of a night out on the grog. Now it's time to explain how to drink alcohol so we stay tidy and have a great night out—with no embarrassing repercussions, a minimal hangover, and feeling refreshed and ready to do it all again the next day.

Step 1 — Before we go out

- We make sure we fill our stomachs with a high-carb food source that can aid in the absorption of alcohol—mashed potatoes, boiled rice, popcorn or a loaf of bread will do the trick nicely.
- We pop a multivitamin pill.
- We have an 'early opener' or two. Downing a few drinks before leaving the house is a good way to settle the nerves

and take the edge off the excitement and anticipation. And it will stop us arriving at the function 'cold' and thereby drinking like demons in our attempt to catch-up. If we're running late and we don't have the time for a few early openers, then we take a couple of 'travellers' for the journey.

Step 2 — On arrival

- We pace ourselves. We want to last the distance and be doing our best work after midnight, at the business end of the evening. We take the first few drinks slowly and allow our body to adjust.

Step 3 — When things are hotting up

- When the party kicks into top gear and we've had a few, we resist the urge to mix our drinks. Mixing drinks, especially the hard stuff, is a sure way to turn ourselves ugly, and an even surer way of ending up with the hang-over from hell.
- We don't, under any circumstance, succumb to peer pressure and be forced into drinking competitions.
- When we've gotten to that point where we feel happy and liberated, then it's just a matter of topping ourselves up every now and again to keep the buzz going. We don't ruin the night by having that one drink too many.
- We understand our limits. It's okay to say, "No thanks, I've had enough for now." Trust me, us blokes get as much respect for our moderation as we do for our excess. To make sure we don't go over our limit, we learn to take note

of the signs that tell us we've had enough. For example, it's time to take a break and hit the bottled water when:

1. We take our mate into a loving hug.
2. We start shadow boxing in the toilet.
3. We think every lady on the dance floor is giving us the eye.
4. We become visibly aroused while dancing with the boss's 55-year-old wife.
5. We reach that point when, though we know what we want to say, somehow our brains are incapable of communicating with our tongues, and we end up talking dribbling gibberish.

Step 4 — When we get home

- Rehydrate, rehydrate, rehydrate! If we drink at least one litre of water before we go to bed, and pop a multivitamin pill, when we wake up the next morning we'll be as fresh as daisies.

Part 7 — Summary and conclusions

Sure, when we're young, it's a rite of passage for us to drink to excess and wake up the next morning face down in a pool of our own vomit, only to discover our mates have shaved off our eyebrows, painted our fingernails, covered our lips in hot pink lipstick and smeared our cohones with Tiger Balm. But as we grow older, getting paralytic is uncool and shows a definite lack of class. An inability to handle our drink could cost us our partner, our mates, our job, our reputation and our health.

A useful anecdote: At 17 years of age, after having had a huge night out, I got home and woke everyone in the house with my puking. Dad got me out of bed at 6 am the next morning and made me mow the lawn. The noise of the lawnmower nearly split my head apart, and the neighbours wanted to kill me. When I finished, my old man simply said, "You wanna be a big man at night, you better learn to be a big man in the morning."

Takeaway learning: The way we handle our drink says a lot about us as men.

Great drinks for a top night out

Every now and again, most of us blokes wouldn't mind a change from our usual brew, but because there are hundreds of alternatives, and because most of us can't be stuffed thinking when we're drinking, more often than not we end up sticking to the devil we know. In the interests of providing us blokes with some viable 'change-ups' from the standard beer, mixed drinks and wines, I have road-tested thousands of alcoholic products and rated them according to:

- Value for money.
- Ability to infuse a non-aggressive, mellow buzz.
- Hangover severity.
- Sexual performance impact.

And using the above criteria, I was able to uncover a few gems. The drinks chosen may be a surprise; they may not be as fashionable or as popular as others on the market, but when it comes to having a good night out, this mob leaves the more commonly purchased 'standards' for dead.

Stout

The Irish are a happy lot; they know how to have a good time. Why? Stout. It does take a little getting used to, with its bitter

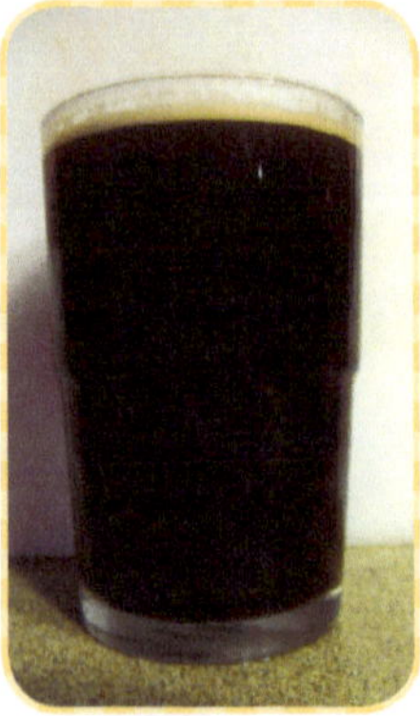

taste and its thickness, but if we give it a go it's sure to bring out the Irish in us. A few of these puppies and we'll be singing Pogues' classics, spinning a few yarns and dancing jigs with the best of them. There's something in stout that brings on a happy buzz, and if you can handle the feeling of swallowing something with the colour and viscosity of sump oil, as well as the next-day-black-poo, then stout is for you.

Cider

Often underrated and overlooked, and commonly mistaken as a girl's drink. Most blokes struggle for alternatives to beer so they hit the spirits when they're ready for a change, only to find the increased alcohol content hits them hard and wipes them out.

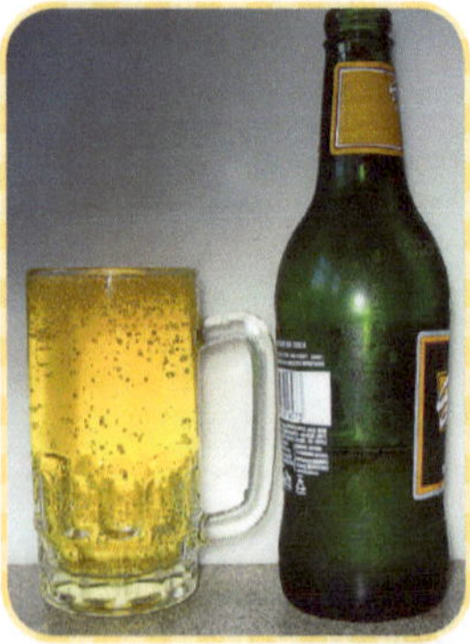

If we've had a gut-full of beer, then why not go the cider option? It's the ideal change-up. It's light, but it packs enough punch to keep us steaming until the early hours without turning us into blithering idiots, leaving us in good shape to have a final crack at picking up, half an hour before closing time, while all the other blokes are face-down in the gutter. Cider is hangover friendly, easy on the pocket, easy on the palate and easy on the waistline. Cider me up, baby!

Ouzo

Ever spent any time on a Greek island? I have, and I'm always amazed at how happy and laid-back the locals are. And when the

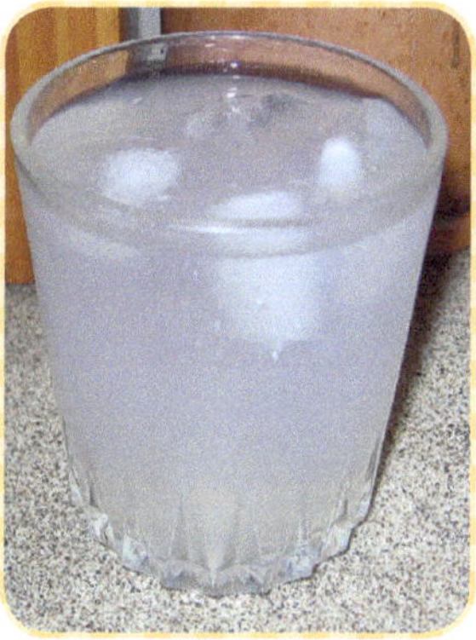

sun goes down, the Greeks know how to party. Why? Ouzo (and maybe the fact that they can kick back all day with a table full of olives and dips and perv on all the half-naked Swedish backpackers). Ouzo mixed with water and a bit of ice is the ideal summer drink. Those who don't like the aniseed taste can mix it with some lemon or grapefruit juice (or raspberry cordial for the sweet toothed). A few ouzos and we'll feel like dancing the Zorba and smashing plates instead of punching on and smashing heads. Oppa!

Vino di Tavolo (Italian table wine)

A real gem of a discovery. Not common, but can be found at the

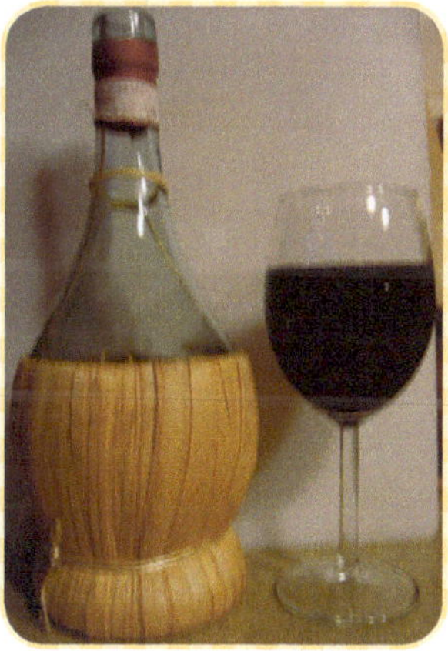

local wine wholesalers or any Guido's backyard distillery. Sounds exotic enough to impress the dinner guests but in reality it's a simple product (made from grapes, smelly feet and not much else) that's cheap as chips. This stuff is low on tannins and preservatives, making it hangover friendly; and best of all, we can drink it by the bucket-load and still have some lead in our pencil at the end of the night when the time comes for a bit of 'amore'. An important cog in the world famous 'Mediterranean diet', table wine is good for the heart and the soul. Think Italian—think fat, happy, healthy and horny. Viva Italia!

Part VIII

Everyday hints and tips

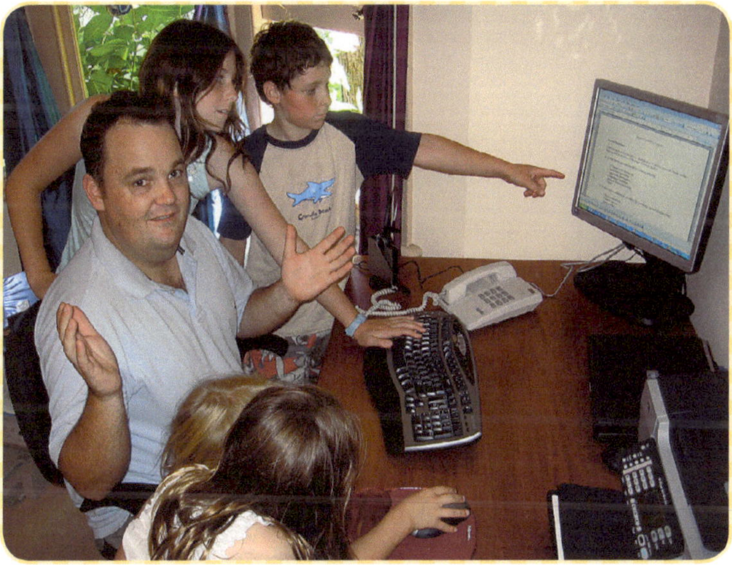

Chapter 40
A man's guide to using a PC

Hell hath no fury like a woman who discovers your porn.

Where once the PC was the domain of brainiac nerds or too-smart-for-their-own-boots kids, nowadays advances in software have made the PC accessible to all men. PCs are powerful tools, with applications that can do everything from keeping household accounts to allowing us to produce our own films. Coupled with the power and scope of the Internet, the PC can bring the world to our doorstep. So given the potential of the PC to make our life easier and more enjoyable, what do most of us use it for:

- Online gambling.
- Exchanging e-mails containing the latest jokes and filth.
- Playing computer games.
- Wasting money buying crap on auction sites.

- Surfing porn.

That's right, us men mostly use PCs for stuff that would cause us great embarrassment if we got caught. And the most common question I get from the lads down at the pub concerning PCs is, "How can I avoid getting caught?"

If we want to avoid getting caught then we must SECURE OUR ENVIRONMENT. Securing our environment doesn't just mean locking our study door when we're partaking in a bit of secret men's business on the Net, it means making sure our 'virtual' and 'real world' environments are safe and intruder-proof.

Securing our virtual environment

Every time we connect to the Internet, we allow others on the World Wide Web to access our personal information, unless we take the proper precautions. If we experience any of the following symptoms when connecting to the Net then there's a good chance our virtual environment is not secure:

- Our homepage is reset without us knowing.
- Our favourites list now includes sites like www.hotnurs-esinpanties.com
- Pop-up boxes advertising all manner of goods and services appear on our screen.
- Web pages keep opening up and we have to keep closing them.

Imagine trying to explain to the missus why www.women-inuniform.com has all of a sudden become our home page. Or explaining to the kids, after they've burst into the study to say goodnight, why there's a web page popping up on our screen, over and over again, with the heading 'ONE MONTH FREE-TRIAL' and a picture of some naked bloke hanging suspended by his testicles while copping a caning from some German chick dressed as a headmistress.

To secure our virtual environment we MUST have up-to-date software that includes:

- A firewall (stops people hacking into our computer).
- A history eraser (erases our history files so no one can tell where we've been).
- A virus checker (prevents computer viruses infecting our system).
- Spyware and Trojan removal program (stops people infecting our computer with software that retrieves our personal details).
- Adware detection program (stops people infecting our computer with software designed to unleash pop-up ads on our screen or redirect our homepage to an advertiser's site).
- Parental control software (stops the kids surfing where they shouldn't be surfing).

These days, for about $100 bucks you can buy an easy-to-install software package that contains all the above components—and it is money well spent.

Handy hint: If you're struggling for a bit of coin, you can get all the protection software you need free from the Internet. Just type 'freeware firewall antivirus' into your search-engine of choice and you'll get tons of sites that offer free downloads.

Securing our real world environment

Okay, now that we've got our virtual environment all set up and well protected, it's time to secure our real world environment. Basically, there are two physical locations where us blokes use our PCs—our home and our place of work.

Securing our home environment

a. **The closed-not-locked technique**
We have our PC set up in a private room (study, home office, shed) with the door closed, not locked. By locking our door we automatically arouse suspicion and guarantee an endless stream of interruptions as the rest of the household do their best to find out why we're being so secretive.

b. **The muffle and scramble**
If we do find ourselves viewing some downloaded erotica, and we're not alone in the house, then we must keep the noises down, or scramble them. We could keep the noises down by hitting the mute button but then we'd miss the all-important sound effects. We could use headphones but then we wouldn't hear approaching footsteps. What we should do is have some music playing in the background—preferably something with explicit lyrics or raunchy sound effects. That way, if our significant other knocks on our door and demands to know what the hell we're doing and why our room sounds like it's hosting a Roman orgy, we can always say, "Just chillin' with a bit of gangsta rap, sweetheart."

c. **The quick switch**

Whatever mischief we're up to on the PC, we make sure we have another web page opened in the background. If our partner does walk in on us, we click on the background web page quick as a flash.

Tip for success: Choose a background web page that is of no interest to the missus—www.sport24x7.com, for example. If she does walk in on you, and you're forced to make the 'quick switch', she's likely to take one look at the web page and say something like, "Sport, huh? Don't you watch enough of that stuff on the TV?" before walking off and leaving you in peace.

d. **The blame it on a mate**

If we're too slow making the 'quick switch' and we get caught drooling over our keyboard while perving on some top-shelf T&A, then we blame it on a mate—a mate our partner knows to be dodgy. Here's an example of the exchange that might take place:

Our partner:	(bursting into room) Dinner's ready.
Us:	(Fumbling mouse) Ughh ...
Our partner:	(Angry) What the hell is that on your screen?
Us:	Um ... It's from Smithy, honey.
Our partner:	You tell that sicko-pervert not to send that smut.
Us:	Gotcha (sigh of relief).

Securing our work environment

BEWARE. Most workplaces now have systems that can track our Internet usage. Most employers turn a blind eye to staff surfing general interest sites, but they do not tolerate staff surfing sexually explicit sites.

Using the Net at work — Rule # 1: Surfing smut is guaranteed to get us the bullet

Workplaces also have sophisticated e-mail filtering systems that stop 'spam' getting through to our in-box. However, the more devious 'spamsters' out there are able to disguise their e-mails in order to bypass security. And these e-mails often contain nasties that can bring the company's network to a grinding halt. We don't want to be the nuff-nuff responsible for crashing the network.

Using the Net at work — Rule # 2: We never open e-mail attachments from strangers

And then there are our mates. We all have mates who are partial to sending the odd 'blue' e-mail to our work e-mail accounts (no matter how many times we tell them not to). Most get picked up by the security systems, but not all, and as soon as we open the attachment—BAM! Up pops a movie that has the boss walking over to our desk wondering what all the commotion is about. If we do receive a saucy e-mail from one of the lads, and we want to have a look-see without risking getting fired, then I suggest we use the MPT security screening system. What is MPT? I hear you ask.

MPT — Meerkat Protection Technique

Meerkats are rodent-type creatures that protect their homes by posting sentries.

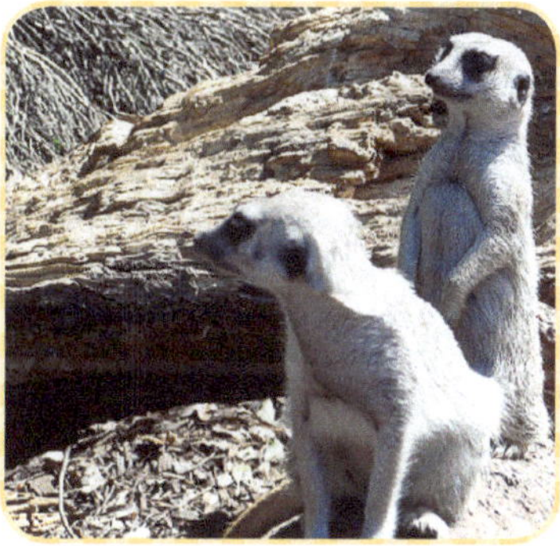

A couple of meerkats standing guard.

On receiving an e-mail we suspect contains highly inappropriate viewing material, we ask a few of our colleagues to stand sentry while we view the material. Should any danger approach (ie, the boss), the sentries then adopt the classic meerkat warning position to alert the viewer of the approaching danger.

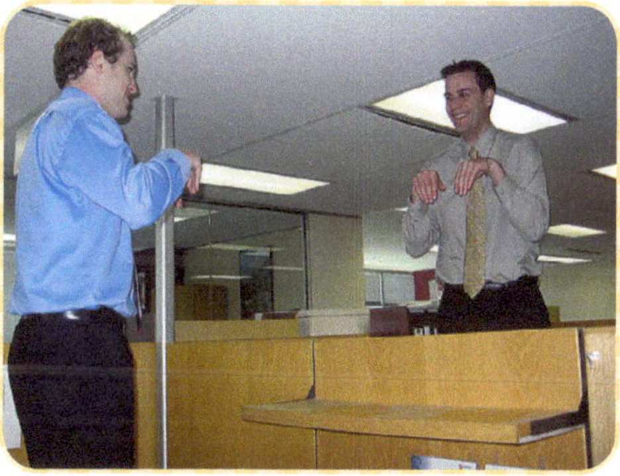

Rob & JC standing sentry for colleague MR X—who is out of shot for reasons of anonymity—while he views a saucy e-mail. Having spotted the boss enter the office, Rob and JC proceed to warn MR X—sitting at the other end of the office—by standing on their desks and adopting the classic meerkat warning pose.

In summary

These days it's almost impossible to surf the Net without being exposed to unsavoury elements. So even if we do use our PC as a tool for productivity, we still need to secure our environment. But if we're using our PC like most blokes use their PC—for pursuits of a dubious nature—then for goodness sakes, we don't do anything illegal and we make sure our environment is well secured.

> *Surfing the Internet without taking the proper precautions is like having unprotected sex—it may be fun for a while, but think of all the nasties you could catch.*
> **(Source: Unknown)**

Chapter 41
How to handle yourself in a punch-on

Let me tell you, standing behind the bar I've seen my fair share of blues, and most of them aren't pretty sights. Gone are the days when two blokes would stand toe-to-toe and sort out their disagreements with a few fisticuffs; where the vanquished walked away with not much more than a bruised ego. Nowadays fights can involve gangs and weapons, and people get hurt—seriously hurt.

We men are taught from a young age that every now and then we need to stand up for ourselves and not be intimidated. Peer pressure amongst us blokes also dictates that any man who backs away is a coward. The problem is, fighting is a skill like any other skill—it requires technique, strength, fitness, and practise. And most of us don't practise our fighting skills because we very rarely need them. So on the odd occasion where we do get the old "You and me outside, buddy" and we're forced to put up our dukes, most of us just charge in, arms flailing, hoping to land a haymaker on the other dude's kisser before he lands one on ours. Fellas, there are other ways.

Why do men punch on?

The first step in avoiding trouble is to understand a man's motives for fighting.

The most common motivators are:

- A skinful of grog.
- Showing off in front of the mates.
- Showing off in front of the girls.
- Retaliation after being punched, bumped or copping an insult.
- Jealousy.

Less common motivators:

- Road rage.
- Too ugly to pick-up so fight to relieve boredom.
- Disputes over material possessions or territory.
- One too many Rocky, Bruce Lee or gladiator movies

Rare motivators:

- To protect someone.
- To stand up for what we believe in.

Developing our sixth sense for trouble

Some men have the ability to sniff trouble as soon as they walk into a room. They're not born with this ability, they've developed it through experience. We too can develop a 'sixth sense' and therefore avoid potential trouble. It's all about reconnaissance work, and here's how to do it:

1. ***Take note of your immediate surrounds***
   Say we've just boarded a plane, and we're belted-up and taxying to the runway. What do the cabin crew get us to do before take off? They get us to check our exits. If we practice doing the same whenever we enter a venue—be it a club, pub, or any other place where alcohol is served—then we'll always know how to escape quickly and, consequently, avoid getting caught up in a fracas.

2. ***Take note of the people around you***
   Footy teams on a night out to celebrate a win = TROUBLE.
   Footy teams on a night out after a loss = EVEN MORE TROUBLE.
   A group of guys drinking Tequila shots = TROUBLE.
   Drunk bikers = SERIOUS TROUBLE.
   A venue where there's only a few single gals and lots of guys = TROUBLE.
   Women who have had an argument with their partner and are looking to get back at them by flirting with other blokes = TROUBLE.
   A group of fans having a drink after watching their team lose = TROUBLE.

Ride the bumps

Whenever we're at a crowded place where alcohol is served, it's more than likely we'll cop a few bumps and knocks. We may be coming back from the bar, or on our way to the toilet, when some well-oiled reveller bumps into us and spills our drinks. Don't react, it's not worth it: a beer costs four bucks but a broken nose can cost hundreds.

Avoid the stares

Most blokes don't like being stared at. Even though our motives for staring may be innocent—the guy may look familiar, for example—more often than not the recipient of the stare is likely to view our prolonged glance as a challenge and, as a result, lock us into a 'stare off', proceeding to hit us with his best dagger-eyes and maybe even a "What are you looking at, shit-for-brains?"

> ***Stare off*** — When two men lock glances, each taking his turn to pump up the intensity of his stare in order to 'stare down' his opponent. Commonly escalates into fisticuffs.

If we do find ourselves locking gazes with some big hairy brute, our best bet is to smile and wave. The big hairy brute is sure to come over, and when he does, we greet him like a long-lost friend. He'll assume we've mistaken him for someone else and move on.

Careful who you're chatting up

If we're out on a mission to pick-up, then we must be careful we don't have the blinkers on and charge in like a bull to a red rag to chat up the first woman who gives us a sideways glance, because that woman may have a partner—and nothing will land us in hot water quicker than chatting up a woman whose boyfriend/hubby is standing at the bar having a quiet drink with a few mates.

Keep in mind, women will check us out (even women with boyfriends). It may be because we look like someone they know, or they may be admiring our fashion sense. Just because a woman looks our way don't mean she's giving us an open invitation to have a crack; we need to look for other signs of interest—a smile, a wink, an arching of the eyebrows.

So if we do spot a lady giving us the eye, we smile at her and see if she smiles back; but before we approach her, we stop, we look around, and we proceed only when there are no signs of significant others—and that way we stay out of trouble.

> ***Word of warning:*** Women generally do not make aggressive first moves. So if some babe appears out of the blue to grab you by the hand and steer you towards the dance floor for a spot of dirty dancing, HANDLE WITH CARE, because she's either been dared by her mates to dance with the first no-hoper she can find or she's trying to make her boyfriend jealous. The former will end in your disappointment, the latter in you copping a knuckle-sandwich.

If you find yourself standing toe-to-toe with a brute

If we've done all we can to avoid trouble but find ourselves in the wrong place at the wrong time, with no backup and some steroid-filled-thick-necked monster standing over the top of us, ready to clobber us into the middle next week—don't panic, there are ways to avoid copping a hiding. The human world is just like the animal world, and in the animal world bluff can be just as effective as bite. Here are a few bluffing techniques we can use to get ourselves out of trouble.

1. **The psycho man**
   We fake an eye twitch and then start howling like a wolf. We jump from foot to foot and then hiss like a snake. We throw a few barks in for good measure and then we start ranting stuff like "The end is nigh, my friend, come with me to the gates of hell." We laugh hysterically and slowly back away. Nine times out of 10 we won't be followed. Trust me, it works. George 'The Animal' Steele was a champion wrestler, and he used to walk around the ring slobbering like a rabid dog and chewing the crap out of the turnbuckles, but not too many messed with our George.

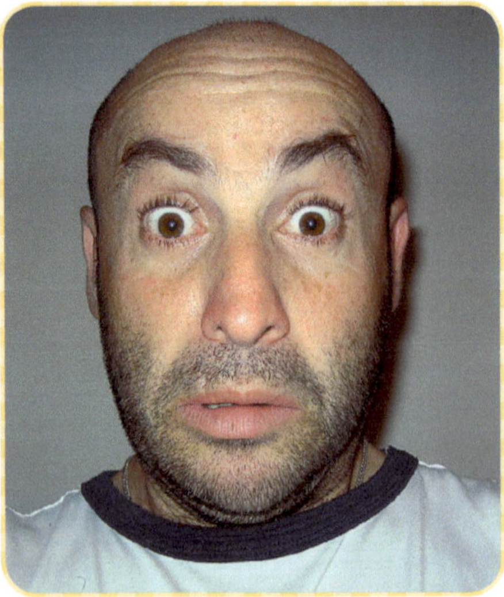

When confronted by a big ugly brute, why look like this when you can look like ...

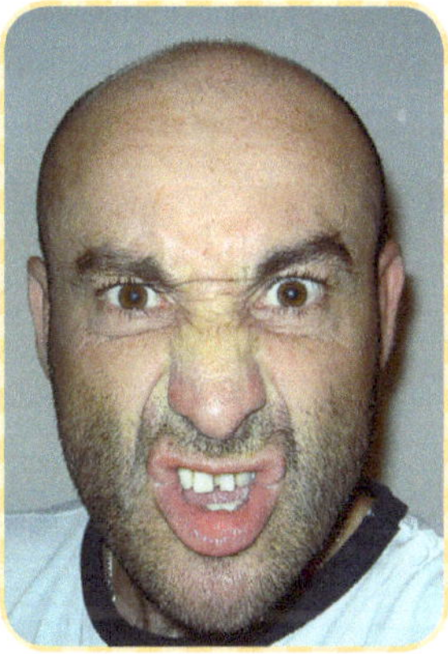

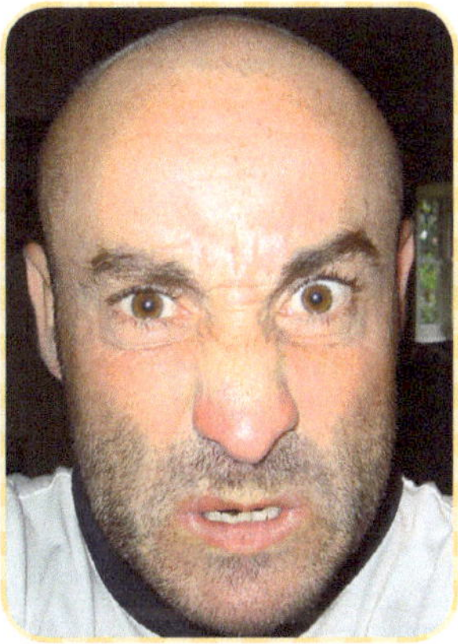

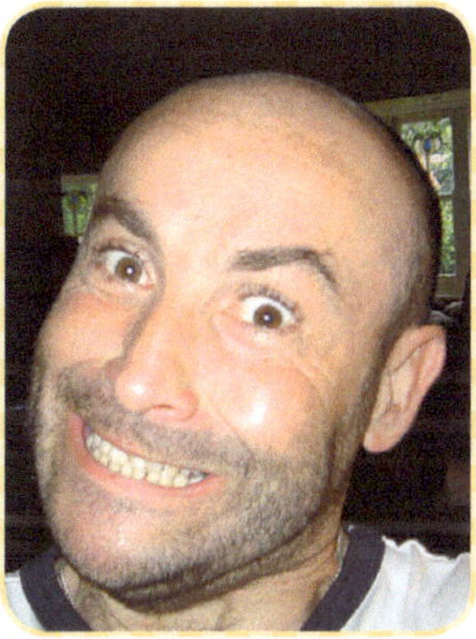

2. **Play dead**

   If we're in the wild and a giant, hairy-arsed grizzly bounds out of the bushes, what do we do? We play dead. Same thing in the urban wild lands. Most blokes won't hit a man who's down, so when confronted with an opponent that is bigger, tougher and meaner than us, we drop like we've been shot and we don't move. This technique may feel a little cowardly, but hell, if it means the other guy decides against belting the stuffing out of us then the embarrassment is worth it.

3. **Fake links to some tough guys**
   Another useful bluffing technique when some nasty hombre is standing over us is to look him in the eye and calmly tell the brute that he can have his fun now but we'll remember his face and we'll catch up with him sooner or later. The brute is likely to laugh in our face, but we don't lose our cool; we throw some names at him that sound like they belong to a group of tough guys, like the mafia or a bikie gang. For example, we could say something like, "I don't want no trouble; I'm not a fighter, but if you beat me up then I'll wait until my cousins, Tony 'The Decapitator' Calabrese and Shotgun Vinnie get out of the big house, and then we'll come a hunting.

If the fists start flying

If we've tried all the above but the big brute standing over us is showing no signs of mercy—in fact, he now has his elbow cocked and his fist clenched in preparation to land the mother of all haymakers smack-bang on our schnoz—then the only thing we can do is try and get the first one in. So we throw as many as we can and hope one lands. If one does, then we don't look surprised and we don't hang around to admire our handiwork—WE RUN!

In summary

Most of us blokes think we can handle ourselves, but the truth is few of us can. Sure, sometimes we get lucky—the other dude is more drunk than us or couldn't punch his way out of a paper bag—but trust me, one day we'll find ourselves staring down some caveman who's been punching-on since he was knee-high to a grasshopper, and we'll end up eating soup out of a straw for months. And that's why it's far better (and healthier) for us average-Joes to dispense with the 'fight first, think later' mentality and adopt an 'avoid first, fight only when there's no other option' way of thinking.

The best way to win a fight is to win it by 50 metres.

Chapter 42
The lost art of the fart

To fart or not to fart — a quandary for the modern man

As kids we run around farting to our heart's content. We fart at school, we fart on our brother's head; we can fart anywhere, anytime, without much fear of retribution. In fact, farting when you're a kid is as much a form of expression as performing in the school play. Nothing much changes as we grow up and move into our bachelor days, but as soon as we start seeing someone regularly or get into a relationship—WHAM! All of a sudden the goal posts shift.

Not all men in relationships are forced to curb their bodily gas expulsions. We've all met the bloke at a social gathering who farts at will while his partner tries her best to look the other way. The type that makes a show of his fart as a way of demonstrating to all the other blokes in the room that no one will ever tell him what he can and can't do. The type who resorts to theatrics with his farts, like lifting a leg or making a face, or adds commentary after letting one rip, such as "I think that one had bones in it".

Regaining our right to fart

Sadly, though, most of us men are fart-pressured as opposed to fart-free. We are forced to get out of a warm bed and into a cold hallway to sound our sphincter-bugle, or go outside, or to another room. Fellas, allow me to let you in on a little secret—our women fart as well.

The thing is, us blokes don't make a big deal out of our partner squeezing one out, because to us it's natural. If we do make a comment, then they act as if their farts smell like a field full of lavender, or they try to act coy and say something like, "It was just a little pop", as if a pop is somehow different to a fart. Bollocks. A fart by any other name still smells as foul.

If we men want to experience some level of fart-freedom, then all we need do is comment every time our partner lets one go, such as "Nice one, sweetie", or "Whoa, there's a bit of activity in the frog pond tonight". The more times we comment, the less likely they'll complain the next time we pass wind.

The art of the fart (how to fart and get away with it)

Unavoidably, throughout our lives, we will find ourselves in situations in which it would be socially unacceptable, not to mention embarrassing, for us to fart. Such situations include dinner parties (particularly when vegetable curry is on the menu), church after a big night out, or when in bed with a girl we're trying hard to impress. But even in these situations it is still possible for us to get some relief; we just have to be smart about it. Here are some techniques that may help:

The quilt lift — For when we need to fart in bed. This technique allows the gas to escape rather than brew under the sheets. Especially good technique for those of us in the early phases of a relationship, or for those who are trying hard to stay in her good books (never, and I repeat never, fart while she's cuddling you).

Quilt lifting technique

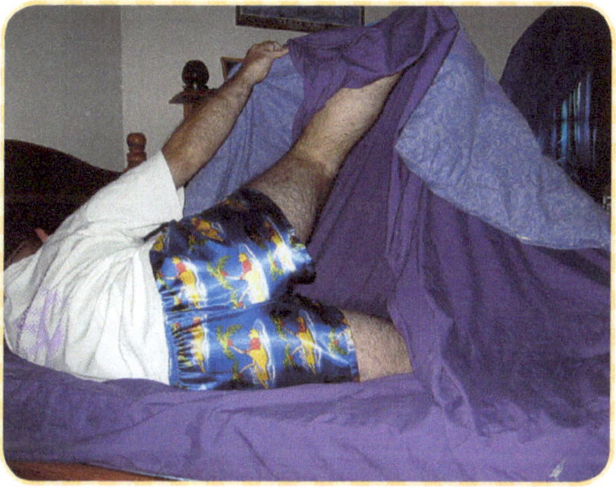

INCORRECT: You want to be subtle, in order to let one rip without her noticing it. High leg extension opens your butt-valve and allows for increased reverb, amplifying the sound of your fart; it also causes maximum quilt displacement—both of which are guaranteed to wake your bed partner.

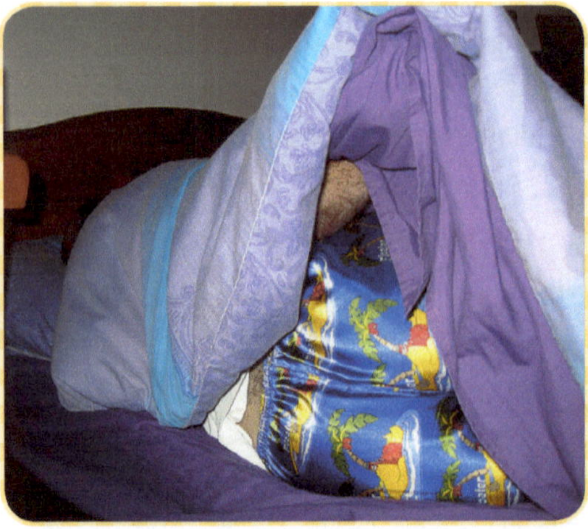

CORRECT: Keep the leg extension to a minimum, in order to minimise quilt displacement, but raise your leg high enough to leave a small opening, allowing the fumes to escape without getting caught up in the sheet. Make sure you keep your cheeks together and squeeze the little beastie out rather than force—this way you'll avoid waking your partner with a ripper.

The blame it on the dog — An oldie but a goodie. If we discover that our hosts have pets, and we desperately need to drop our guts, then we make our way over to the dog and we release our gas while we're giving it a vigorous pat. Mission accomplished. When using this technique, however, it is important to remember that we must let our gas escape as silently as possible. It's no good trying to blame the dog after letting go a fart that that's loud enough to shatter crystal.

The sneeze and fart — We have no control over our bodies when we sneeze. So if we've got a ripper ready to launch, we sneeze and fart at the same time, and no one will be able to point the finger.

The stepped in poo — Another classic. If we've let go a jock-clinger—one of those farts that follows us around like an orphaned duckling—and someone makes a comment, then we innocently check the soles of our shoes before turning to everyone (making sure we look suitably embarrassed) and telling them we must have stepped on a dog-grenade.

The drop-your-guts and run — Great for when there's no one else around to blame for our gaseous emission. Let it out and then run for the hills.

Chapter 43
Social etiquette for the average Joe

Don't worry, I'm not going to talk about which knife we ought to use when cutting up our steak, because quite frankly, who cares? What I will talk about are the etiquette challenges that concern the average bloke on the street.

Toilet etiquette

There's way too much talk about whether us blokes should leave the toilet seat up or down after we've done our business. It's no good putting the seat back down if we've peed all over it and hit the walls and floor with the resulting spray. Let's not get ahead of ourselves, first things first—we concentrate on our aim, not the position of the toilet seat. Women can live with a man who leaves the toilet seat up, but a man who can't aim is a different story.

We aim to keep this toilet clean, your aim will help.
(Source: A sign above the toilet at the pub where I work)

Table etiquette

The fact that we don't know our dessert spoon from our soup spoon and we use the tablecloth to wipe our mouth doesn't necessarily make us an uncultured simpleton. What will make people turn up their nose is if we do the following:

The loud belch

No doubt, there's not much to rival the feeling of downing a beer and then letting loose a satisfied burp, and in some cultures it is expected. But if we want to get further than a first date, or we want our wives to invite us to their work dinners, then we must learn to exercise some self-control. The next time we feel the need to burp, we try closing our mouths and letting the gas escape through our nose—it may singe a few nostril hairs but we're unlikely to scare the hell out of our date with a burp that would wake the dead. And, for those of us with kids, never encourage the little tykes by acknowledging their belches with a "Bravo, tiger" or a "That's my boy", otherwise we may find most of our invites printed with the words:

No kids.

Double-dipping

Nothing gets up people's goat more than a bloke who slams his rice-cracker into a jar of salsa, takes a bite, and then returns the slobbery half-eaten rice-cracker to the salsa jar for another scoop. He may as well have just spat in the dip. To eliminate this problem, we simply shove all of what we're dipping into our mouths at one time.

Chewing with mouth open and noisy eating

No one wants to see the contents of our food being churned in our mouths like cement in a cement mixer. Nor do they want to hear us eating our dinner. Unfortunately, once we get into the habit of mouth-open-noisy-eating, it's tough to address the problem because our mouth muscles become used to holding our jaws open while we chew. Our partners can shout at us to keep our mouths closed while we eat till they're blue in the face, but we're still likely to lapse, unless—we use a bit of electro-shock-therapy. Sounds harsh but it's the only way.

> ***Tip for success:*** Get yourself down to the electronics store and buy some gear that will enable you to get rigged up for a mild electric charge. Get your partner or a trusted mate to sit with you while you eat, and every time you start chewing like a mule with a mouthful of hay—zap! Two or three sessions and problem solved.

The starving animal routine

Us blokes like to launch into our food and swallow it as fast as we possibly can, without talking or breathing. The 'have-food-must-eat' mentality is a survival instinct harking back to our caveman days, and it's a tough one to get under control. Common behavioural patterns of the 'have-food-must-eat' instinct are:

- Hunching over the plate as if protecting it from someone trying to steal the food.
- Launching into the food as soon as it hits the table.
- Knocking over cups and jugs and leaning over other guests to get to the choicest cut of meat.
- Inability to converse while food is on the table.

- Fighting with the kids over the last bread roll.

If we're at home, then we can probably get away with acting like a pig at swill; but if we're at someone else's table, then we slow down, look up and breathe.

Socialising etiquette

If we're attending a function solo, or with the partner, then we try to avoid doing the following:

- Heading for the nearest TV to watch the sport.
- Scratching our nuts.
- Picking our nose (especially the 'pick, roll and flick' routine).
- If it's a function where finger-food is being passed around, we don't hover around the serving staff picking off food at will, and we don't hip and shoulder other guests in a frantic attempt to get to the waiter with the calamari rings that we love so much.
- If there's a tab running, we don't use up half the tab ourselves by ordering the most expensive beers and spirits, or stay at the bar downing one beer after another out of fear that the tab may run out.
- If it's a dinner party we're attending, then we bring a bottle of wine for the host and enough grog for ourselves. We drink what we bring and not everyone else's more expensive imported stuff. We leave anything we don't drink with the host, otherwise we'll be seen as a tight-arse.
- AND for goodness sakes, if we're attending a function with the significant other, we don't abandon her at first

sight of our mates. AND we don't get the first drink without getting her one as well. We get her a drink, and then we piss off and join our mates. Everyone's happy.

In summary

Us blokes needn't worry if we know bugger-all about wines, cheeses and which bread roll is ours—the one on the left or the right? If we cover the etiquette basics and be ourselves, then people will find us easy to get along with and a refreshing change from all the toffy-nosed snobs they usually associate with. And when it comes time for us to leave the dinner party or function, our hosts are sure to say, "I like having that Joe character around for dinner; he's got no class but he's a nice bloke." And after all, isn't that what we all strive to be?

The Final Word

So you've got to the end—congrats. Thanks for taking the time out to read the book. Hopefully you'll have picked up some tips and tricks to help you become happier and healthier. Just in case you've forgotten all that you've read, here are some guiding principles to help you become the man you always wanted to be.

The 10 guiding principles for successful manhood

1. A dog is not your best friend, your penis is. Learn to love it!
2. Be happy with yourself and people will learn to love you, no matter how ugly you are.
3. The happiest men are those with nothing to prove.
4. Look after your mates and they'll look after you.
5. A bit of exercise won't kill you.
6. Clothes don't make the man, attitude does.
7. Successful relationships are all about love and avoidance.

8. Sex is like golf—it's impossible to keep up with all the modern trends and innovations, but take some time to learn from the pros and your handicap will come down in no time.
9. Learn to handle your grog and you'll be well respected.
10. Women are different to men. Spend some time talking to them instead of just thinking about what they'd look like in skimpy lingerie, and you'll be a wiser man for it.

And finally, and most important of all:

Don't take life too seriously, have a laugh!

Also by Joe Novella

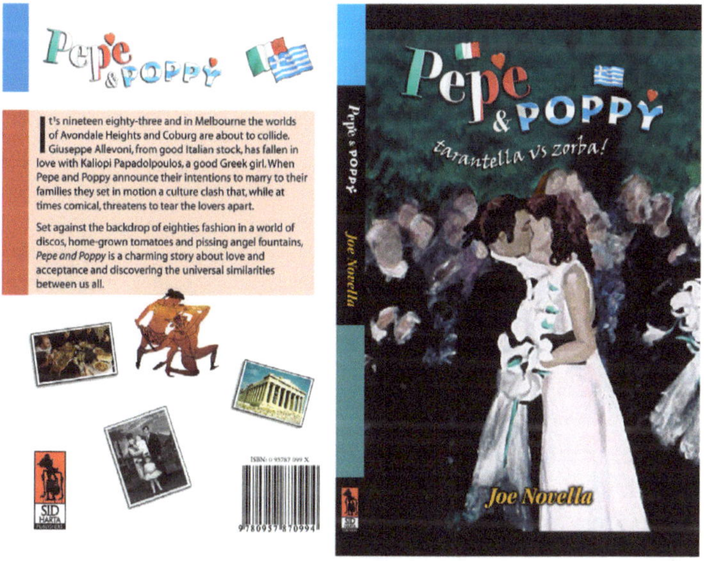

Pepe & Poppy
It's nineteen eighty-three and in Melbourne the worlds of Avondale Heights and Coburg are about to collide. Giuseppe Allevoni, from good Italian stock, has fallen in love with Kaliopi Papadolpoulos, a good Greek girl. When Pepe and Poppy announce their intentions to marry to their families they set in motion a culture clash that, while at times comical, threatens to tear the lovers apart.
Set against the backdrop of eighties fashion in a world of discos, home-grown tomatoes and pissing angel fountains, Pepe and Poppy is a charming story about love and acceptance and discovering the universal similarities between us all.
SID HARTA
Pepe & Poppy
Joe Novella
Pepe & POPPY
tarantella vs zorba!
Joe Novella

Please visit my website at

www.joenovella.com

for news on my latest projects, to give me some feedback on current projects, or just to say hi.

www.ingramcontent.com/pod-product-compliance
Lightning Source LLC
Chambersburg PA
CBHW040928030426
42334CB00002B/5
* 9 7 8 0 9 8 7 1 8 4 4 3 6 *